THE
5-DAY
DIET

Lose weight, supercharge your
energy and boost your health

PATRICK HOLFORD

piatkus

PIATKUS

First published in Great Britain in 2020 by Piatkus

1 3 5 7 9 10 8 6 4 2

Copyright © 2020 Patrick Holford

The moral right of the author has been asserted.

A CIP catalogue record for this book
is available from the British Library.

ISBN 978-0-349-42579-5

Typeset in Minion by M Rules
Printed and bound in Great Britain by
Clays Ltd., Elcograf S.p.A.

Papers used by Piatkus are from well-managed forests
and other responsible sources.

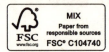

Piatkus
An imprint of
Little, Brown Book Group
Carmelite House
50 Victoria Embankment
London EC4Y 0DZ

An Hachette UK Company
www.hachette.co.uk

www.littlebrown.co.uk

Contents

Part 3

Transitioning to a Low-GL Diet

Acknowledgements

I am indebted to Professor Valter Longo, who first pioneered the fasting-mimicking diet, and to Jerome Burne, co-author of *The Hybrid Diet*, for sparking my interest in all things ketogenic. I would also like to thank Marcelle Dubruel and Jo Muncaster, my co-conspirators in our 5-Day Hybrid Fast Detox Retreats in the Black Mountains of Wales. Together we have found out what works for people, and what doesn't, to come up with what I believe to be the winning formula for rapid health renewal. Jo has tweaked the recipes until they are perfectly delicious within the complex nutritional requirements for this diet to work. I am also most grateful for the support and innovation of Ros Lincoln and Donna Gambazza and their team for developing the support products for the 5-Day Diet.

Important Note

This book is intended to provide helpful information. It should not be taken as medical advice. Neither the author nor the publisher accepts liability for readers who choose to self-prescribe. If you have a specific medical condition or are on any medication consult your GP before beginning the diet.

Guide to Abbreviations and Measures

1 gram (g) = 1,000 milligrams (mg) = 1,000,000 micrograms (mcg or μg). Most vitamins are measured in milligrams or micrograms. Vitamins A, D and E are also measured in International Units (iu) – a measurement designed to standardise the different forms of these vitamins, which have different potencies.

1mcg of retinol (mcg RE) = 3.3iu of vitamin A (RE = retinol equivalents)
1mcg RE of beta-carotene = 6mcg
100iu of vitamin D = 2.5mcg
100iu of vitamin E = 67mg
1 pound (lb) = 16 ounces (oz)
2.2lb = 1 kilogram (kg)

In this book, for simplicity, I use 'calories' in place of kilocalories (kcal). There are 9 calories in 1g of fat, and 4 calories in 1g of protein or carbohydrate.

Introduction – Five Days to a New You

A discovery of massive importance has been made: how to reset, reboot and renew your cells in five days while, at the same time, kick-starting a weight-loss diet and losing extra pounds easily. It is based on the fact that the body under certain circumstances of lower calories and protein (but no animal protein) triggers a self-healing process called 'autophagy', which literally means 'self-eating'. Autophagy repairs and replaces damaged cell parts, including the energy-generating factories, which are called mitochondria. This is especially important if you have experienced a gradual reduction in energy or have health issues niggling away at your full experience of life.

In addition, you'll find that this 5-Day Diet normalises blood sugar levels, reducing cravings for both sugar and alcohol, normalises blood pressure, cholesterol and blood fats (triglycerides), and reduces pain and inflammation. This makes it excellent for those with diabetes (with some provisos explained on page 7), heart disease or arthritis wishing to make a quantum leap towards health.

All this adds up to a potentially profound anti-ageing effect, with better production of stem cells, the foundation cells from which we develop all new cells, from skin cells to brain cells.

It is not a diet for life, but specifically for five days, after which I recommend that you follow my low-GL, or slow-carb, way of eating to continue with weight loss and then to adopt it as a lifestyle maintenance diet. The low-GL diet is easy to do anywhere, even in restaurants, if you order wisely. This should become your way of life, with the 5-Day Diet used as a reboot every now and again in much the same way that you put your car in for a service. It's also a great way to kick-start weight loss if you've been gradually gaining weight or need to trim down for the summer, after Christmas, or to fit into all those clothes you used to wear. Generally, I recommend that healthy people follow my 5-Day Diet four times a year, and that people who have specific health issues that they wish to reverse do it once a month for at least four months, as this has been shown to reset health to a higher level; for example, animals with autoimmune disease have reversed their condition with four cycles (more on this in Chapter 1).

In Part 1 I explain the theory: why the diet works and how to trigger autophagy without fasting completely; what ketones are and how ketosis works (see opposite for a brief description); the process of detoxifying your body; and supporting healthy digestion and elimination when a low calorie intake inevitably means eating less fibre.

In Part 2 I'll explain how to do it: the drinks, foods, recommended supplements, exercises and also how to monitor your progress, including 'bio-hacking' (measuring how your body is responding via ketones in your breath or a pinprick blood test for your glucose and ketone levels), for those who choose to.

In Part 3 I explain how to transition to the low-GL lifestyle diet.

Ketones and ketosis

For fuel, your cells can either burn glucose or ketones made from fat. When you switch from primarily running on glucose to running on ketones your blood, urine and breath levels of ketones will go up. This is called ketosis. (I explain this crucial element of the diet in detail on pages 18–19.)

The discovery of the health benefits of autophagy was originally made by studying what happens in total fasting, but now we know that you can get an even better result by not completely fasting, but by following a strict and very precise diet, plus taking supplements that are high in autophagy triggers. What these are and how they work, as well as the inner workings of my 5-Day Diet, will all be explained in this book so that you can follow it and experience the immediate rewards for yourself.

I became fascinated by this topic when I was researching *The Hybrid Diet*, co-authored with award-winning medical journalist Jerome Burne, and the tales of transformation achieved in animals and humans, including the reversal of both type-2 diabetes and autoimmune type-1 diabetes (in animals), as well as rapid weight loss, energy gain and reduction in pain with all hard measures of vital statistics (from cholesterol to inflammatory markers) in humans. I'll explain how autophagy works in Chapter 2, as well outlining the foods and nutrients that act as autophagy triggers, which are all included in the 5-Day Diet, and how to exclude all the foods and lifestyle elements that act as autophagy blockers.

As I will explain in Chapter 1, this diet is based on my trial run in 2019. I took 14 volunteers aged from 34 to 74 on a retreat in Wales for seven days, giving them the last two days to 'transition' to my slow-carb maintenance diet explained in Part 3, and it is the inspiration for this book. The volunteers started with a variety of aches, pains and conditions such as diabetes, and I wanted to see how they would respond to my 5-Day Diet followed by my slow-carb lifestyle diet and whether their health benefited. I also followed the diet with them. I was delighted to find that there was a weight loss of 34.2kg (75lb) across 14 people – an average of 5lb (2.5kg) – and their health markers improved. Furthermore, people were able to follow the very low-calorie part of the diet comfortably and reported that they did not feel excessively hungry but soon enjoyed the benefits from the diet, which continued to grow as they followed the low-carb phase that followed.

Supercharge your energy

Something I also experienced after the retreat, as did many others, was an undeniable supercharge of energy and clarity of mind in the weeks after the 5-Day Diet. Here's what the volunteers reported: 'Energy now better than normal, mental acuity – brighter', 'In all honesty I feel 100 per cent better', 'But I feel tighter and pretty irresistible !' 'I haven't experienced *any* sugar temptation, which I would usually find difficult to resist', 'I am very focused and find my mind is very clear and organised', 'Sleep is great since retreat', 'I am feeling extra-good: mood great, energy great', 'I feel in control and very relaxed about my food. I haven't felt like snacking in the evenings, which is new for me.' In all, you really feel as if your whole energy metabolism has been given a reboot – a supercharge.

This is, of course, really exciting, with maximum benefit for minimum effort, but there is another side to this, which is now being explored in a number of research studies relating to 'irreversible' autoimmune diseases, from type-1 diabetes to rheumatoid arthritis, neurological disorders from Parkinson's to dementia, and also certain cancers, especially glioblastoma brain cancers. Dr Thomas Seyfried at Harvard Medical School is using ketogenic diets with great results for these kinds of brain cancers.[1] (It's too early to say if this approach is beneficial for all cancers in all stages, but certainly to starve cancer cells of sugar seems to be a universally good idea.) The lifetime risk of cancer has quickly escalated from less than one in ten to one in three in the past 40 years, and that means that a set of factors (not genes, since they haven't changed) is forcing our cells to tip into a diseased cancer state. The idea that we could reset our cells and immune system to tip back to a healthy metabolic state is perhaps the most exciting new frontier in nutritional medicine today. By following the 5-Day Diet with my low-GL diet as your baseline way of eating you'll be making some important steps towards protecting yourself from disease.

I'll fill you in on the latest findings in Chapter 1 so that you can see who is more likely to benefit from this approach, the most researched version of which is called the fasting-mimicking diet, devised by Professor Valter Longo of the University of Southern California. My 5-Day Diet goes two steps further, pulling out all the stops to trigger autophagy and also to support detoxification. It is also easier in terms of the level of hunger and withdrawal effects and tastier with our tailor-made recipes.

Going hybrid

I'm also going to show you what to eat before and after the five days, which involves switching from burning fat for fuel to eating slow carbs. The 5-Day Diet is 'hybrid' because it involves five days on very low-carb, high-fat foods, triggering ketosis, whereby your energy cells switch from burning glucose to ketones derived from fat, followed by going on to my low-GL diet, which means that your body will switch back to running on slow carbs. This low-GL diet has a weight-loss element and a lifestyle element, so you can move easily from one to the other when you have reached your weight-loss goal. This becomes your baseline diet for life. Those who have read *The Hybrid Diet* will understand the value of switching, from time to time, from a low-GL/slow-carb diet to a high-fat, very low-carb ketogenic diet. It seems that doing this 5-Day Diet once a month if you're overweight or not that healthy, or once a quarter if you are, is the fastest way to improve your health and to protect yourself against future ill-health.

A modified fast

The 5-Day Diet is a modified fast because you'll be eating about 800 calories a day, which is the lowest you can go without feeling really hungry, but it is low enough to trigger autophagy, your cellular system reboot. This low-calorie phase is supplemented with specific nutrients. I'll be explaining exactly how you can boost this important process in your body by using specific calorie-free nutrients in supplements that trigger autophagy.

Total fasting leads to loss of muscle mass and that's something you don't want, especially if you are older. By doing a small amount of aerobic exercise, as explained in Chapter 6, you'll maintain your muscle mass. The beneficial results, including weight loss, are also surprisingly fast. You will be amazed at how much better you feel in a very short space of time.

Rapid detox

When you go into ketosis, burning off excess body fat, you also release stored toxins, because the body dumps toxins that it can't get rid of fast enough into storage in body fat. As a consequence, you can feel worse after a couple of days when you fast. It's called the 'healing crisis', but I think it's just a crisis because, on a total fast, you are not taking in any nutrients to support the liver, which has to work hard to process released toxins for elimination in the urine; however, by including specific nutrients, especially antioxidants that support liver detoxification (as explained in Chapter 8) you won't suffer at all. This is all taken care of in the 5-Day Diet.

Who shouldn't do the diet?

The diet is fine for people with type-2 diabetes who are either drug-free or who control their diabetes with metformin alone, but not for those people who need medical supervision and dosage adjustment of other drugs that they are taking – the danger being blood sugar dips.

I'd caution against this approach for anyone significantly underweight, where losing a few extra pounds would be a concern. For those who don't need to lose weight, you might lose

2–3kg (4 to 7lb), mainly from belly fat. This diet is designed to preserve lean body mass, if followed together with the specified exercises in Chapter 6.

If you suffer from a specific disease, check with your doctor as to whether there would be any contraindications with the medication you're on. I am not claiming that this diet prevents, reverses or treats any disease as such.

If you do experience any adverse symptoms check the Troubleshooting section in Chapter 10. I also have a private group on Facebook, as part of my 100% Health Club, which I check almost every day (see Resources), where you can seek help with basic practical questions and suggestions if you get stuck or suffer minor symptoms, but this does not constitute medical supervision. If in doubt, please speak to your doctor or primary healthcare provider.

Wishing you the best of health,

Patrick Holford

Part 1

The Theory – Why the 5-Day Diet Works

The 5-Day Diet is not just a low-calorie diet to lose weight. It is specifically designed to trigger a self-repair process, called autophagy, which renews and rejuvenates your cells, reboots your metabolism and detoxifies your body. This part explains why it works.

Chapter 1

The 5-Day Benefits of Fasting, without Fasting

The benefits of complete water-fasts, where nothing is eaten for several days, are well established in scientific studies, with minimum risk of significant adverse effects.[1] The trouble is that only the brave are willing to do it. Yet now we have a growing body of proof that you don't have to completely fast to get the same benefits, and you might even get *more* by a five-consecutive-day low-calorie fast designed to trigger autophagy, the body's cellular repair process (which I will explain in the next chapter).

Some people fast for one day a week, others eat fewer calories twice a week on a 5:2 diet and others do 18:6, meaning 18 hours without eating, usually by having an early dinner, skipping breakfast, and then eating a late lunch. There are many other variations of intermittent fasting. All these have their merits and reasonable evidence, or at least logic, to support them. All will have the potential to briefly trigger autophagy and nudge your metabolism away from glucose, made from carbs, towards ketones, made from fat, including burning your own body fat.

Yet I do not believe that they are nearly as effective as five consecutive days of fewer calories, with not too much protein, and consuming food and drink that is specifically designed to trigger autophagy, which is the key to the ability of fasting to transform your health, rejuvenate your cells and switch you out of a disease process.

A leader in the pioneering edge of the five-day diet approach, as I explained in the Introduction, is Professor Valter Longo, a biochemist and gerontologist at the University of Southern California. It was Longo's research that inspired Michael Mosley to try a basic version of the 5:2 diet for his TV programme *Eat, Fast and Live Longer*. The rest is diet-book history. But Professor Longo himself much prefers five consecutive days, perhaps once a month for the less well, or once a quarter for the healthy. His research, and that by others, suggests that this five-day fasting-mimicking diet has the potential to:

- Reverse autoimmune disease.

- Reduce cancer risk, and possibly help to shrink tumours for some cancers (but not all).

- Repair cells and generate new, healthy mitochondria, which means more energy.

- Burn fat fast.

- Reduce inflammation.

- Enhance brain function, and help to prevent, arrest and possibly reverse some neurodegenerative diseases.

- Reverse diabetes and cardiovascular disease.

You can think of this five-day process much like a system reboot. By taking your foot off the carb accelerator, your body will slow down your metabolism and switch to burning ketones, then go into self-repair mode. It's like putting your body in for a full service.

Longo's research has shown that this five-day approach improves many biomarkers for ageing, diabetes, heart disease and cancer, with no adverse effects. One study involving 71 people found a broad range of health improvements illustrated by changes in significant markers such as weight, blood pressure, blood glucose levels and total cholesterol.[2] However, 'What was remarkable', says Longo, 'was that those who were well – with low blood pressure, low triglycerides and low-glucose – saw no change. That's very different from what happens with simple calorie restriction, which just keeps driving your markers down, whatever they are.'

He says that his diet also 'may help people to become more metabolically flexible. First, they switch to fat burning and start oxidising fatty acids for energy and then they switch back to more carbohydrates and glucose. So, you get accustomed to using both glucose and fatty acids as sources of energy.'

Longo's fasting-mimicking diet is a five-day fast, during which participants eat between 800 and 1,000 calories per day, but with the same ratio of carbs, protein and fat (5–10, 20–25 and 70–80 per cent, respectively) as they would on a ketogenic diet.

It even has the potential to regrow parts of damaged organs and bring defunct insulin-producing beta-cells back to life. Some of the most interesting studies, hinting at reversal of auto-immune disease and cell renewal, have only been carried out in cell and animal subjects at this point, but there are human studies underway, which will be published in the next few years.

My 5-Day Diet is a low-carb, low-calorie, fasting-mimicking diet that pulls out all the stops in order to trigger autophagy, burn fat and detoxify the body. It is ketogenic, meaning that your body switches from burning glucose (carbs) to burning ketones, made from fat, including your own body fat. While other popular high-fat low-carb ketogenic diets, the original being Atkins, have posted great weight loss results, they are too high in protein, especially animal protein, and calories to trigger the benefits of fasting or 'fasting-mimicking diets'.

The 5-Day Diet trial

To test the 5-Day Diet I took 14 volunteers on a retreat in Wales. Some had diabetes and some had autoimmune disease. Most were overweight with a variety of common health problems ranging from arthritic aches and pains, to poor sleep, low energy, mood dips, asthma, depression, anxiety and stress. In other words, they were a good cross-section of people from 34 to 74 years old, 3 men and 11 women. They all trialled this 5-Day Diet followed by two days eating the low-GL (low-glycaemic load) diet. I also followed it myself.

Exercise was restricted to mild cardio exercise: a short walk to raise one's heartbeat just enough to activate the major muscles. The reason for this will become clear, but briefly, full-on resistance or muscle-building exercise switches off autophagy.

We measured weight, body fat, ketones, glucose and various health measures, from energy levels to pain, as well as hunger. I wanted to know what was happening close up.

I had three main concerns that could scupper the success of this experimental diet. The first was how long it would take to get people's metabolism to switch from primarily burning glucose (our body's preferred fuel) to burning ketones and to go into ketosis, the stage that precipitates autophagy, and switches your body into fat-burning mode. The convention is that it takes two to seven days to switch into ketosis, and the less healthy you are the longer it would take. That could be a problem because I wanted my volunteers to be in ketosis for five days. To achieve this, everyone had a low-carb lunch the day before, with dinner at 7pm, followed by effectively an 18-hour carb fast, with lunch at 1pm on Day 1. In the morning, however, they had my special Hybrid Fast Latté (see page 61), containing C8 oil, which is the oil, derived from coconut, from which the body can make ketones quickly (see pages 21–23). The blood and breath tests showed that everyone was in ketosis within 24 hours. It had worked.

My second concern was that people would have the often-reported keto flu: feeling achy, groggy and irritable after a day or two as the body's metabolism switches to running on ketones. I know from experience with clients that many people quit a ketogenic diet because of this initial suffering. I had some ideas about how to avoid this and what to do if you do experience specific sugar withdrawal symptoms, and I explain these on page 109, and it, too, worked. No one reported keto-flu symptoms or felt like giving up. One woman, Emmanuelle from France, had a mild headache on Day 2, and felt weak for a couple of hours but that soon resolved and she started to feel fabulous, with much more mental clarity, by the next day. Most people were reporting better energy, a calmer mood and better sleep by Days

2 and 3. I asked people to rate their health concerns out of ten with, for example, ten out of ten for energy being the best and zero out of ten being the worst. Emmanuelle's brain fog went from 3/10 to 8/10. For the group, overall energy went from 5/10 to 7.5/10. Many people reported having better sleep, from 5/10 to 9/10 as a group average, and better mental health, memory and reduced anxiety, with the average score going from 4/10 to 8/10. Aches and pains also reduced dramatically for some people. Jodie found that she could 'move and walk more' and is on her way to being 'pain-free'. Tina's asthma almost disappeared. Blood sugar levels for the group normalised quickly, even among the diabetics, to levels they had never recorded since being diagnosed.

My other concern was hunger. After all, 800 calories is not much to eat in a day, but the exact sequence of foods, and the special fibres added to prevent constipation, meant that no one reported hunger. 'You don't feel as if you're being deprived in any shape or form, and you come away feeling a million bucks,' said Lynn from South Africa.

In terms of weight, if you believe that it's all about calories, five days on 800 calories should have caused about 10kg (22lb) weight loss for the group as a whole. In other words, a little under 1kg (2lb) each.

Now, there's a bit of a cheat when people report weight loss in the first week of a no-carb diet, because you first have to burn off all the stored glucose, which is held in the liver and muscles as glycogen: glucose plus water. You can easily lose 2kg (4lb) just in water as you go into ketosis. That's why people impressively lose weight in the first week of the Atkins diet. But that water weight loss will come back as the body restores glycogen reserves, which is what it does as soon as you come out of ketosis and back to a diet with carbs.

We were careful, therefore, to measure the final weight loss not after five days in ketosis but after reloading with carbs on the sixth and seventh days of eating the low-GL diet, containing slow carbs, and no longer 800 calories. This is the kind of diet you can live on as your maintenance diet: a lifestyle choice.

The total weight loss for the group was 34.2kg (75lb) across 14 people – an average of 5lb (2.5kg). That's more than double what you'd expect from the calorie reduction. People were burning fat, not muscle, and something magical was happening to their metabolism. I've never seen results like it, both in the short term and one month later. Most people who needed to lose weight had lost 7kg (14lb) a month later.

I lost over 2 stone (14kg/31lb) and all my belly fat, with my body-fat percentage going from 30 per cent down to 16 per cent, which is ideal, over the three months that I have been following this 5-Day Diet, once a month. Now in my sixties I have found it increasingly easy to gain weight, and harder to lose it, but now I know how to rapidly get back to my ideal weight and body-fat percentage with ease. It's as if my metabolism has reset itself.

As I described in the Introduction, the volunteers reported a variety of positive effects including greater energy and clarity of mind in the weeks following the 5-Day Diet and the transition to the lifestyle low-GL diet.

Can autoimmune diseases be reversed?

Autoimmune diseases (which include rheumatoid arthritis, multiple sclerosis, Hashimoto's thyroid disease, systemic lupus erythamatosus (SLE), Crohn's disease, ulcerative colitis and type-1 diabetes) are very much on the increase.[3] They all involve the immune system wrongly targeting something in your body, be it your joints, nerves, thyroid, gut or, as in the case of type-1 diabetes, the cells that make insulin.

One study that received a lot of attention put mice with type-1 diabetes, which were thus unable to make insulin, on the 5-Day Diet, then they had nine days off, then back on the diet, completing four cycles. The researchers found that *during* the five days there is cell *repair*, but *after* the five days there is cell *renewal*. This strategy, then, put the animals through a repair–growth–repair–growth cycle four times.

Type-1 diabetes is an autoimmune disease because the immune system selectively kills off all insulin-producing cells, hence those people with type-1 diabetes have to inject insulin for life. It is considered irreversible. The mice started to make insulin, thus reversing their type-1 diabetes.[4]

Another study with mice looked at inflammatory bowel disease. This group of conditions includes ulcerative colitis and Crohn's disease, both of which are autoimmune diseases. The control treatment followed water-only fasting. In this case it was four days on the fasting-mimicking diet, or water-only fast, then nine days off, repeated four times.

Both groups had reduced intestinal inflammation and improved gut microbiota, but only the fasting-mimicking diet reversed the intestinal damage, so it was more effective than a water fast, not just by improving symptoms but also reversing the disease and repairing the damage.[5]

Upgrade your brain

The other area where this approach is likely to have major benefits is in giving your brain cells an upgrade. Nerve cells and brain cells are both neurons. Unlike other cells – muscle cells for example – they cannot directly burn fat. They have to have a direct supply of one of two fuels, either glucose or ketones, which are made in the liver from certain kinds of fat, specifically one called C8, which I'll talk about in a minute. These two fuels – glucose or ketones – are like five-star fuel for the brain. Brain cells need a direct supply of either pure glucose or ketones, much like a hybrid car can either run on petrol or electricity.

Which fuel do neurons prefer? The answer is ketones, if given the choice. Ketones help to make new neurons[6] which is why a newborn baby's brain is largely using ketones, derived from fat, to build the brain rapidly. Many people, especially later in life, and more especially those with a neurodegenerative disease such as dementia or Parkinson's, might have neurons whose glucose engine is furred up and unable to produce enough energy or brain power, and therefore they are chugging along in the brain equivalent of second gear. (Those with epilepsy and, perhaps, multiple sclerosis, and some people diagnosed with chronic fatigue syndrome, might also have similar problems.)

Switching fuels by greatly limiting carbs and increasing fats that readily turn into ketones might help these cells to recover. Moreover, in addition to providing emergency energy supplies, autophagy (the cell repair process triggered by ketosis) seems to offer some protection against brain disorders, including Parkinson's disease. Neurons use a lot more energy than other cells, so the brain cells' mitochondria, their energy factories, need to be especially efficient. It's possible that inadequate or malfunctioning autophagy is also a factor in the development of Alzheimer's, given that the condition is characterised by a build-up of plaque and other waste products in the brain.[7]

C8 oil and dementia

A recent study looked at 52 people with pre-dementia.[8] It measured how well neurons were functioning and determined that the participants' brain cells were not fully firing, in other words they would be experiencing effectively a lack of brain energy, which would be experienced as poor concentration, memory and ability to process information.

The participants were given either two tablespoons (30g) of C8 oil, which is part of my 5-Day Diet, or a placebo, and changes in their cognitive function were measured. In those that were given the C8 oil, the half-firing neurons came back to life. Brain ketone metabolism increased by 230 per cent, indicating that their brain cells were switching to using ketones as fuel, and the more this was happening the more cognitive improvements occurred.

Unlike other fats, C8 oil goes straight to the liver via the portal vein, thus not requiring all the digestion that other fats require. The ketones then enter the blood and are taken up, as an energy source, by the cells' mitochondria.

In this study the participants weren't on a very low-carb ketogenic diet, thus they were still eating carbs, but clearly they still received a significant brain benefit. The researchers excluded diabetics from the study so they weren't looking at people with abnormal glucose metabolism; however, they *were* people suffering with cognitive decline.

Can a ketogenic diet be of benefit for people with Parkinson's and epilepsy?

A study on people with Parkinson's found that those who were put on a high-fat ketogenic diet had a 41 per cent reduction in shaking, compared to 11 per cent on a low-fat diet.[9] There's also a potential benefit for those with chronic fatigue syndrome.[10]

Epilepsy, for example, has been successfully treated in both children and adults with a high-fat ketogenic diet since the 1920s, often halving the frequency of fits.[11]

You might not have any of these diseases, but will you nevertheless benefit from a good supply of ketones to your brain? Although I know of no definitive studies yet, many people report a jump in concentration and focus following, and during, the 5-Day Diet. In our experiment, the average self-reported mental-health score went from 4 out of 10 to 8 out of 10 – a doubling in self-reported mental health, including clarity of mind and reduction in anxiety.

It is highly likely that much of these benefits are down to two things:

1. Switching from burning glucose to burning ketones.

2. Switching on autophagy, the cellular repair process.

Exactly what triggers autophagy is explained in the next chapter.

Before we get into the wonders of autophagy, which is really how fasting works, it's important to know that you get a lot more ketone production in the liver from eating very specific fats, not just following any old high-fat diet. Selecting these ketogenic fats is a critical part of the 5-Day Diet.

The fast way to ketosis

Ketones are made from a type of fat called medium-chain triglycerides (MCTs). Recently there has been a big increase in sales of oils high in MCTs, which are generally sold as MCT oil, although the amount and kind of MCTs can vary a lot. (Also gaining in popularity are ketone salts and pure synthetic ketones, although these are yet to clear the EU Novel Foods regulations, so they are not yet available in Europe.)

MCTs are found in high concentrations in both coconut and palm oil, as well as dairy butter, and they convert into ketones in the liver. Coconut oil is 60 per cent MCTs. I avoid palm oil, however, unless it is produced from undeniably sustainable sources, since the destruction of the rainforest to grow palm oil on an industrial scale is the reason the orangutan is threatened with extinction.

Fats, including MCTs, are made of carbon chains of differing lengths. Stearic acid, the main fat in meat, has 17 carbon chains (C17), whereas olive oil is mainly 14 chains (C14). Anything below 12 chains (C12) and above 6 chains (C6) is classified as 'medium chain' or MCT. The gut bacteria can synthesise very short-chain fats such as butyric acid, which is C4. There's also some C4 in goat's cheese.

The different MCTs are:

- C6 – caproic acid triglyceride

- C8 – caprylic acid triglyceride (also called tricaprylin)

- C10 – capric acid triglyceride

- C12 – lauric acid triglyceride

Of these, pure C8 most readily converts into ketones, raising ketones in the blood far more than just coconut oil or so-called MCT oil. In a study that gave volunteers either a control substance, with no MCTs, coconut oil, C8 or C10 oil coconut oil was little better than the control, whereas C8 oil raised ketone levels almost five times higher (see opposite).

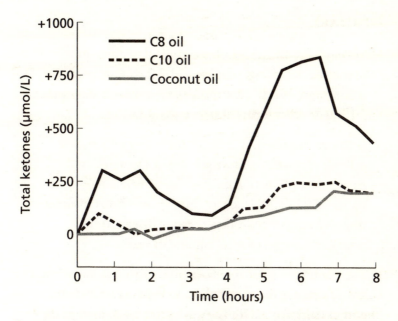

Data from Vandenberghe et al, *Current Developments in Nutrition, 2017*

Some better quality MCT oils combine C8 and C10 but, even so, this is much less effective than pure C8 oil; for example, C8 oil raises ketones roughly four times higher than C10.[12] The long and short of it is that nothing raises ketones better than C8 oil, and neither MCT oil nor coconut oil is a substitute.

The vast superiority of C8 oil to coconut oil is not surprising when you realise it is the C8 oil in coconut that actually makes the ketones. Although coconut oil is 60 per cent MCTs, only 12 per cent of MCTs is C8. That means that only 7 per cent of coconut oil is C8. Therefore, you would have to consume ten times as much coconut oil to get the same amount of C8 as pure C8 oil, which is a lot of extra fat and calories for the body to process. Pure C8 oil is part of your Hybrid Fast Latté 'breakfast' during the 5-Day Diet (see Chapter 5).

SUMMARY

- Through existing research we know that a five-day reduced-calorie, high-fat, low-carb, fasting-mimicking diet is more effective for transforming health than water fasting or other forms of intermittent fasting.

- It has many potential benefits, including anti-ageing cellular renewal, rapid weight loss, an increase in energy, brain function enhancement, reversal of metabolic diseases (such as diabetes and heart disease), improvement of neurodegenerative diseases and potential reversal of autoimmune diseases.

- The main reason for these benefits is through switching away from glucose metabolism to ketone metabolism, and switching on autophagy, which is the subject of the next chapter.

Chapter 2

Autophagy – How to Reboot, Repair and Rejuvenate Your Body

We now know that the miracle of fasting is largely attributed to autophagy. In fact, in 2016 the Nobel Prize in Medicine or Physiology was awarded to the Japanese researcher Yoshinori Ohsumi, a cell biologist at the Tokyo Institute of Technology's Institute of Innovative Research for his work on unravelling the miracle of autophagy.

Manufacturing protein and generating energy in the body create as much waste and junk on the nano-scale within our cells as they do on the macro-scale in our global environment. Therefore, an efficient rubbish-removal system for each of our 37 trillion cells is essential if our bodies are to continue functioning properly.

Autophagy, which, as we have seen, literally means 'self-eating', hoovers up dead and damaged proteins as well as disposing of burnt-out mitochondria – those energy factories contained in our cells. All this waste matter is combined with enzymes within the lysosome (see opposite), the equivalent of a recycling plant, that recycles most of it into fresh energy supplies and the raw materials that will be used to create new proteins, from which new and rejuvenated cells are made.

When you start the 5-Day Diet, the sharp drop in carbohydrates immediately triggers the starvation response. As the levels of glucose and insulin in the blood start to decline, the body switches on autophagy and starts its rubbish-collection and recycling process.

How autophagy works

Millions of microscopic structures called 'phagophores' act rather like bin lorries, collecting the accumulated rubbish. These ever-expanding trucks trundle around the body's cells, engulfing dead or damaged proteins, bacteria, viruses and exhausted mitochondria as they go. Next, they transport all the waste products and foreign bodies they have collected to the lysosome – a large bubble filled with enzymes that dissolve proteins into their constituent amino acids. When the crisis is over, and you go on to my low-GL slow-carb diet, growth resumes and the recycled amino acids are once again turned into new proteins. That's when cellular renewal kicks in big time, and this is why there's a second layer of benefits to the 5-Day Diet, such as increased mental and physical energy experienced in the weeks after you've completed the five days.

Autophagy

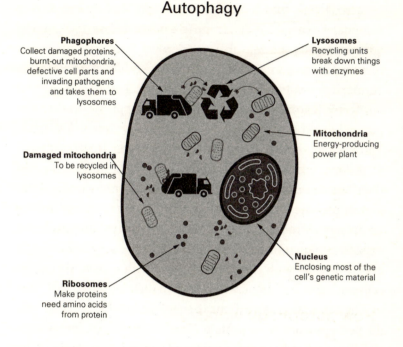

Phagophores
Collect damaged proteins,
burnt-out mitochondria,
defective cell parts and
invading pathogens
and takes them to
lysosomes

Lysosomes
Recycling units
break down things
with enzymes

Mitochondria
Energy-producing
power plant

Damaged mitochondria
To be recycled in
lysosomes

Nucleus
Enclosing most of the
cell's genetic material

Ribosomes
Make proteins
need amino acids
from protein

As early as the 1930s, it was discovered that animals that are fed 30 per cent less than normal are very healthy, with good metabolic markers, such as low blood pressure, low glucose and insulin, and a healthy body mass index. Now we know that this 'lean eating' encourages more autophagy.

The mitochondria mop up oxidants, harmful waste products that are released during energy production. As we age, however, this system starts to deteriorate, and DNA can be damaged at an increasingly rapid rate as a result. Fortunately, autophagy weeds out the most damaged mitochondria before they can do too much harm. This is just one of the reasons why it's so important to kick-start the repair process through autophagy on a regular basis.[1]

Another reason for encouraging the repair process is that

cancerous cells find it harder to multiply and spread during autophagy. This is because phagophores (those bin lorries) quickly identify the defective cells, hoover them up, and deposit them in the lysosome, where they are broken down. In addition, 'Autophagy limits oxidative stress, chronic tissue damage, and oncogenic [cancer cell] signalling, which suppresses cancer initiation'[2] to quote a study in a *Clinical Cancer Research* journal. That's all good news if you want to stay cancer-free, but there's a caution if you have cancer. Unfortunately, if a tumour is given the chance to establish itself, the balance of power might shift, as it will be able to use the amino acids that are produced during autophagy as fuel to meet its very high-energy demands and expand into surrounding territory.[3] I therefore urge caution with experimenting with this diet for those with cancer. (If cancer cells are starved of sugar, which is often their preferred fuel, they will hunt for other ways to make energy, much like normal cells do, perhaps from fat or protein. That is why you can't really say that there is *one diet* that is right for all cancers at any point in the treatment process.) Please check with your doctor or oncologist.

Damaged mitochondria and its link to ill health

Recent research suggests that a wide range of illnesses might be linked to damaged mitochondria that have lost the ability to burn fat or glucose efficiently.[4] A case in point is chronic fatigue syndrome, in which energy production is obviously compromised.[5] As such, it is imperative to keep clearing out the worst-performing mitochondria through autophagy.

Autophagy itself tends to become less efficient as we get older, however, probably because the body's lysosomes lose some of their ability to recycle amino acids. That's why the 5-Day Diet is so beneficial: because it pushes the body into autophagy on a much more regular basis and therefore forces the lysosomes to keep working. This is one reason why this kind of approach is a promising treatment for chronic fatigue syndrome, which is experienced as low energy.[6]

How to trigger autophagy – your cellular self-repair

Fasting, or starvation, however, is not the only way to trigger autophagy, although it is the most important. For this reason the 5-Day Diet limits calories to about 800 calories a day. Furthermore, in the last five years, I have found that many of the nutrients and foods that I've been recommending over the years for other health-promoting reasons also directly trigger autophagy. These autophagy trigger foods and nutrients include:

- A high-fat, ketogenic diet (provided it is low in protein and calories)

- C8 oil – such as Ketofast

- HCA – from garcinia cambogia, a type of tamarind

- Alpha-lipoic acid – a key antioxidant

- High-dose vitamin C

- Zinc, found richly in seeds, shellfish and fish

- Magnesium, in seeds, beans and greens

- Niacin (vitamin B3)

- Oily fish, rich in the key DHA fatty acid in omega-3 fish oils

- Polyphenol-rich and sirtuin-activator foods (which turn on genes that activate autophagy), such as:

  Olives and top-quality olive oil high in oleuropein and oleocanthal, such as Drop of Life (see Resources)

  Spinach, kale, broccoli, cabbage, watercress and rocket – the sulforanes and kaempferol[7] are the active ingredients

  Mushrooms – especially shiitake mushrooms

  Blackcurrants, blueberries and blackberries

  Turmeric – it's the curcumin[8] that is important

  Ginger, due to a compound called 6-shogaol

  Cacao, due to its theobromine content[9]

  Cinnamon[10]

  Coffee/caffeine/theophylline, green tea, hibiscus, mint, berberine (in Goldenseal tea), bergamot (in Earl Grey tea)

You have to take in these foods and nutrients *without increasing* your carb content, or allowing your protein intake to go too high. All of the above are an inherent part of the 5-Day Diet; mostly you will find them in the foods and drinks, although it will be necessary to take some as supplements in order to have sufficient quantities to trigger autophagy while food intake is low. Some foods that have ingredients that trigger autophagy, such as red grapes, are excluded because their sugar content, or the calories needed to get the autophagy effect, would have an overall *anti-autophagy* effect. It's a fine line, a nutritional juggling act, but don't worry because all this is taken care of. All you need to do is follow the instructions.

What blocks autophagy?

These are autophagy blockers that switch off cellular self-repair:

- High calories

- High carbs, especially sugar and fructose (fruit sugar)

- High protein, especially meat and dairy

- Increased IGF-1 levels (insulin-like growth factor)

- Any dairy product, which promotes IGF-1

- Resistance or strength training; for example, body building

As is often the case when a whole new scientific area opens up, much of the research starts on cells and animals, so we have to be careful not to assume that the same thing will happen with humans. But it can take years before human trials are carried out, so you might have to take a call on it, especially when the logic is strong. That's what I've done in the 5-Day Diet. It's the state of the art for switching on autophagy.

Nutrients that trigger autophagy

An oral administration of HCA, the active ingredient in garcinia cambogia (a type of tamarind), when given to mice for two days, triggered autophagy comparable to that induced by water-only fasting starvation.[11] This single food compound had as great an autophagy effect as fasting. Since we already know that prolonged treatment with HCA, in both animals and humans, is known to cause significant weight loss, and this effect is not explained away by reduced food intake, neither does it have adverse effects in the amounts needed for benefit, it's a no-brainer to take it for triggering autophagy. HCA helps you to burn food for energy rather than putting it into storage as fat. It is one of my favourite weight-loss aids (as you will see in Chapter 8) and I strongly recommend that you take it three times a day on the 5-Day Diet.

I believe we will find a number of antioxidants that help to trigger autophagy as they, too, are part of the body's clean-up squad. Alpha-lipoic acid, which I supplement every day as part of my daily antioxidant formula, has a dozen good trials clearly showing its ability to switch on autophagy, but none have as yet been carried out in humans. Animals supplementing with alpha-lipoic acid, however, do live longer.

Vitamin C also triggers autophagy.[12] Many degenerative neurological diseases, such as Alzheimer's, show raised levels of damaged proteins. Autophagy clears these away. According to a cell study, 'Supplementation of the culture medium with physiological concentrations of vitamin C did not affect protein synthesis, but did increase the rate of (abnormal) protein degradation by lysosomes. Vitamin C accelerated degradation by autophagic pathways.'[13] This means that normal protein manufacture, necessary for healthy muscles, went on regardless, but damaged proteins got cleared away.

We do also have some human clinical evidence for autophagy triggers: for example, a study on elderly Chinese people who were given 2g a day of DHA (the brain-building omega-3 fat found in oily fish) found it improved both cognitive function and autophagy of damaged amyloid plaque.[14] In other words, the DHA helped to trigger a clean-up of damaged proteins in the brain, which are linked to Alzheimer's dementia.

SUMMARY

If you put all this together, the best strategy for triggering autophagy, and consequently cellular repair, is:

- To follow a high-fat, low-carb, low-protein, and low-calorie diet (circa 800 calories) for five consecutive days.

- To be dairy- and meat-free, with a direct source of DHA from seaweed and oily fish – mackerel, salmon, tuna, anchovies and fish roe (such as taramasalata) – caviar is by far the richest source of DHA.[15]

- To take C8 oil.

- Supplementing HCA, alpha-lipoic acid and high-dose vitamin C, zinc and DHA.

- To eat olives, olive oil, kale, broccoli, cabbage, spinach, watercress and rocket.

- To drink coffee, Earl Grey or green tea, hibiscus, bergamot or peppermint tea.

  All these are included in the 5-Day Diet.

Chapter 3

Detox Support for Your Cellular Clean-Up

Although eating the right food and getting sufficient nutrients is one side of the coin, detoxification is the other. Detoxification is a natural process carried out by the body to remove toxins produced from everyday living. Most substances we consume – including food, water and air – contain toxins as well as nutrients and generate toxic by-products as we make use of them. Think of these as the exhaust fumes created by burning carbs, fat and protein, the latter being used day in and day out to make new cellular material. Oxygen, for example, turns into carbon dioxide (CO_2), which gets exhaled in the breath. When following the 5-Day Diet you'll also be releasing toxins that are stored in fat, which is where the body dumps toxins that it can't easily transform and remove. Most of these toxins have to be detoxified by the liver, which acts like a clearing house, able to recognise millions of potentially harmful chemicals and transform them into something harmless or prepare them for elimination. Your liver is the chemical brain of your body – recycling, regenerating and detoxifying in order to maintain your health.

External – or 'exo' – toxins, ranging from exhaust fumes to pesticides and industrial pollutants, represent a smaller part of what the liver has to deal with; and even more toxins are made within the body as a by-product of processing what you eat, drink and breathe. These internally created – or 'endo' – toxins have to be disarmed in just the same way as the exo-toxins. Whether a substance is bad for you depends as much on your ability to detoxify it as its inherent toxic properties. Those people with multiple food sensitivities, for example, are eating the same food as healthy people, but they have lost that detoxification potential. If this is the case for you, it's important to regain your capacity to detoxify so that you can feel better and increase your energy and ability to deal with physical and mental stress.

Measuring your detox potential

If you are experiencing multiple allergies or food intolerances, frequent headaches, sensitivity to chemicals and environmental pollutants, chronic digestive problems, muscle aches and inflammatory conditions, there's a good chance that you have exceeded your capacity to detoxify. This can be a huge additional stress on your body, so regaining your detoxification ability is an essential part of feeling better and building greater health resilience. You can get an instant impression of your detox potential by completing the questionnaire overleaf, which lists the symptoms associated with poor detoxification. Score yourself now, and then retake the questionnaire a week after you've completed the 5-Day Diet.

Questionnaire: Check your detox potential

	Yes	No
1. Do you often suffer from headaches or migraines?	☐	☐
2. Do you sometimes have watery or itchy eyes, or swollen, red or sticky eyelids?	☐	☐
3. Do you have dark circles under your eyes?	☐	☐
4. Do you sometimes have itchy ears, earache, ear infections, drainage from the ears or ringing in the ears?	☐	☐
5. Do you often suffer from excessive mucus, a stuffy nose or sinus problems?	☐	☐
6. Do you suffer from acne, skin rashes or hives?	☐	☐
7. Do you sweat a lot and have a strong body odour?	☐	☐
8. Do you sometimes have joint or muscle aches or pains?	☐	☐
9. Do you have a sluggish metabolism and find it hard to lose weight, or are you underweight and find it hard to gain weight?	☐	☐
10. Do you often suffer from frequent or urgent urination?	☐	☐

	Yes	No
11. Do you suffer from nausea or vomiting?	☐	☐
12. Do you often have a bitter taste in your mouth or a furry tongue?	☐	☐
13. Do you have a strong reaction to alcohol?	☐	☐
14. Do you suffer from bloating?	☐	☐
15. Does coffee leave you feeling jittery or unwell?	☐	☐

Score 1 for each 'yes' answer.

Total score: ☐

Score

8 or more
If you answer yes to eight or more questions, you need to improve your detox potential.

4–7
If you answer yes to between four and seven questions, you are beginning to show signs of poor detoxification and need to improve your detox potential.

Fewer than 4
If you answer yes to fewer than four questions, you are unlikely to have a problem with detoxification.

Detoxification – a two-step process

The main mechanisms for detoxification are carried out by your liver and involve a complex set of chemical pathways that have the ability to recycle toxic chemicals and turn them into harmless ones, in a process known as 'biotransformation'. Each pathway consists of a series of enzyme reactions, and each enzyme is dependent on a number of nutrients that, step-by-step, make your internal world safe to live in. Detoxification can be split into two stages, known as Phase 1 and Phase 2.

Phase 1

The first phase is akin to getting your rubbish ready for collection. It doesn't actually eliminate anything but just prepares it for elimination, making it easier to pick up; fat-soluble toxins, for example, which you'll be releasing as you burn fat, become more soluble. Phase 1 is carried out by a series of enzymes called P450 enzymes. The more toxins you're exposed to, the faster these enzymes must work to pile up the rubbish ready for collection. Harmful substances that get Phase 1 working hard include caffeine, alcohol, pollutants, cigarette smoke, exhaust fumes, high-protein diets, preservatives such as benzoates, organophosphate fertilisers, paint fumes, damaged trans fats, steroid hormones and charcoal-barbecued meat.

How the liver detoxifies

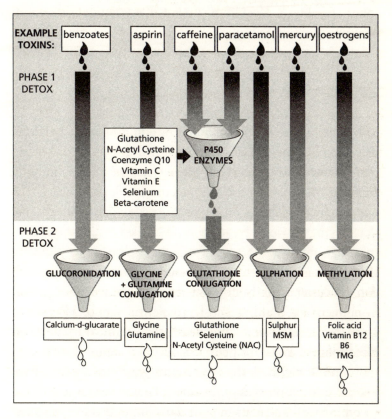

The Phase 1 P450 enzymes depend on antioxidant nutrients to detoxify the damaging substances. These include glutathione, n-acetyl cysteine, coenzyme Q10, vitamins C and E, selenium and beta-carotene – although B vitamins, flavonoids and phospholipids are also important. Although you'll be eating foods that contain many of these nutrients during the 5-Day Diet, you won't be getting enough to maximise the support your liver will need, and it will then be working overtime to clear the released toxins. For this reason I recommend taking specific supplements containing these nutrients, and they can be found in one all-round antioxidant formula. I'll let you know exactly what to take in Chapter 8. Most important of all is vitamin C, so as well as supplementing 1 gram a day, I'll be recommending you take a daily drink that includes powdered vitamin C (ascorbic acid).

Phase 2

This second phase is more about building up than breaking down. According to Dr Sidney Baker, an expert in the chemistry of detoxification, about 80 per cent of all the building that the body does is for the purposes of detoxification. The end-products of Phase 1 are transformed by 'sticking' specific detoxifying nutrients on to them. It's called conjugation, as in marriage; for example, some toxins have glutathione joined to them (this is called glutathione conjugation) to proceed with detoxification. This is how we detoxify paracetamol (acetaminophen) for example and in cases of overdose a person is given glutathione, or its precursor (the chemical from which glutathione can be formed) – n-acetyl cysteine (NAC) – to mop up the highly destructive toxins generated by the Phase 1 detoxification process of this drug. Glutathione is one of the recommended nutrients in your daily antioxidant supplement and it is also found richly in onions and garlic, which are part of the recommended foods in the 5-Day Diet.

Other toxins have sulphur stuck to them in a process called sulfation. (This is the fate of many steroid hormones, neurotransmitters and, once again, paracetamol.) The sulphur comes directly from food. Garlic, onions and eggs, for example, are good sources of sulphur-containing amino acids such as methionine and cysteine – so if you have a lack of these in your diet, you've got a problem. These foods are included in the 5-Day Diet. Other toxins have carbon compounds, called methyl groups, stuck to them (this is called methylation and depends on B vitamins, especially B6, B12 and folic acid). Lead and arsenic are detoxified in this way. So too is adrenalin. That is why your recommended support supplements (see Chapter 8) provide optimal amounts of all the B vitamins that support methylation, while the diet provides nutrient-rich foods. Vitamin B12 is especially important to supplement, as it's only found in animal foods, which are very much restricted in the 5-Day Diet since too much of them turns off autophagy.

Too many toxins or not enough nutrients?

These two detoxifying pathways work together. If one is overloaded, a toxin can be processed by another pathway known as glucuronidation. Cruciferous vegetables and turmeric contain compounds that support this pathway and are important foods in the 5-Day Diet.

Once the back-up systems are overloaded, however, either because you're taking in too many toxins or your body has run out of the nutrients needed to make the detox pathways work, your body is unable to clear the toxins, which can then damage and disrupt just about every system of the body, affecting the nervous system, hormone balance, muscles and joints, digestion and immunity. This can be a factor in chronic fatigue syndrome in which a person often feels worse after eating or physical exertion because they are unable to detoxify even the normal endotoxins properly.

Many low-calorie diets and fasts don't factor this in, so, although a person might start to look better as they lose weight, they actually feel worse. During the five days of the diet you will have stopped taking in toxic substances and you will also have increased your intake of liver-support nutrients, thus having an opportunity to regain detox resilience in terms of improved liver function. This is probably the main reason I have very few people reporting adverse symptoms as their body's metabolism transitions from burning glucose to breaking down fat and burning ketones. Detoxification overload is probably a major reason for the so-called keto flu mentioned on page 15, as the body starts to break down fat when starved of glucose – fat that has been the dumping ground for toxins.

Summary

The 5-Day Diet provides all the nutrients, both in the foods and in the support supplements, to maximise the liver's ability to eliminate toxins that might be released as you switch over to burning fat. The foods, drinks and supplements combined are a necessary part of this detox support.

Chapter 4

Digestive Support for Healthy Elimination

A common cause of toxic overload is problems in the digestive tract, as this is the major route by which the body eliminates toxic material. Your ten-metre-long digestive tract stretches from your mouth to your anus, with a series of corrugations, called villi, in the small intestines, designed to maximise the surface area. If ironed out flat, your digestive tract would cover a small football pitch! This huge surface area forms a barrier between the 100 tonnes or so of food we consume in a lifetime and our inner world – in other words, all that's inside us on the other side of the wafer-thin epithelial cells that line the digestive tract. Only certain digested molecules are allowed through this barrier into your bloodstream via a specific selection process, which is policed by the immune system. These epithelial cells that make up the gut wall work hard to transport nutrients from the food you eat into your body and they regenerate every four days.

In the 5-Day Diet you'll be eating an extremely clean diet, and thus you will have the chance to literally rebuild a healthy digestive tract; however, with fewer calories and virtually no carbs it becomes extremely challenging – in fact, actually impossible – to get enough fibre for healthy elimination. Even on higher calorie ketogenic diets constipation is one of the most commonly reported adverse effects. (If you google it, you'll find over a million pages on this topic.)

The right kind of fibre

Contrary to popular opinion, high-fibre diets don't necessarily relieve constipation unless the fibre is soluble, which means that the fibres absorb water. The richest food sources of soluble fibre are oats and chia seeds. That is why oats make good porridge, because they absorb the moisture, swell up and become creamy, while chia, when soaked, expands to absorb ten times its volume in water.

Psyllium is another choice, but the soluble fibre par excellence is konjac fibre, which is high in glucomannan. Glucomannan fibre is the most water-absorbent fibre of all, absorbing 100 times its weight in water.

When you include glucomannan fibre in your meal you feel fuller after the meal, plus it lowers the GL of the meal by slowing down the release of sugars in foods and thus helps to stabilise blood sugar. (Read more about the glycaemic load, and why it is important, in the box on pages 54–55.) Glucomannan is one of the very few natural substances that is allowed to carry an

EU health claim for weight loss if accompanied with a lower calorie diet.

Glucomannan also helps to promote healthy bowel movements, relieving constipation and improving gut ecology, according to a Chinese study of constipated adults.[1] It is the lighter, bulkier, more watery faecal matter that moves through the digestive tract, propelled by the peristaltic (pushing) motion of the musculature of the gut, that relieves constipation. We should go to the toilet twice a day, without straining, with loosely formed stools.

Smooth digestion with fibre and vitamin C

The other nutrient that helps to move things along in the digestive tract is vitamin C. According to EU law, supplements containing vitamin C have to give a warning that large amounts can cause loose bowels. Of course, this is a benefit for many and it certainly helps to keep things moving along during the 5-Day Diet.

During the 5-Day Diet I'll be asking you to make a drink in a 500ml bottle, three times a day, that contains vitamin C and glucomannan fibre. This means that in addition to any herbal teas, you'll be drinking 1.5 litres of water, which is, in itself, a help for healthy bowels, detoxification and elimination.

Into each 500ml water bottle you'll be adding half a measured teaspoon of glucomannan fibre and half a level teaspoon of vitamin C (ascorbic acid) powder. Glucomannan has no flavour as such, whereas pure ascorbic acid is tart. For this reason, many vitamin C powders contain sugar. These cannot be used on the 5-Day Diet. I recommend, therefore, ImmuneC High Potency powder (see Resources), which also contains berry extracts but no sugar, adding flavour to the water. It also contains ascorbates, which are an alkaline form of vitamin C attached to important detox nutrients, such as magnesium. (If you cannot get this, pure ascorbic acid powder is the next best thing.) This will give you the optimal amount of vitamin C and glucomannan for digestive elimination and detoxification, when added to water. If you find this too tart, you could try adding adding a teaspoon of Blueberry Active, a concentrate of blueberries available in health food stores.

I recommend that you load up your 500ml bottle, ideally transparent, three times a day – in the morning, after lunch and after dinner – and you should make sure that you drink the entire bottle before the next meal. This will give you a steady supply of water, as well as the sensation of being full. Alternatively, you could fill a 2-litre bottle with 1.5 litres of water, plus the glucomannan and vitamin C and drink a third three times a day.

Vitamin C dissolves, whereas glucomannan absorbs water. You need to shake the bottle, not just when you add the powders, but several times over the first five to ten minutes to fully disperse the ingredients and absorb the water and prevent clumping. This is also why I prefer glucomannan to psyllium husks, which have a tendency to clump and have actually made some people's constipation worse. In the US and Canada there is a fibre called PGX (see Resources), which includes glucomannan, and this can be used in the same way as glucomannan fibre.

The best herb teas and herbs for healthy digestion

In addition to drinking the water described above, you need to drink at least two cups of herbal tea, choosing from those that also trigger autophagy but are not too sweet. These include:

Black Earl Grey tea*

Ginger

Goldenseal tea

Green tea with bergamot*

Hibiscus

Peppermint

Turmeric

* These two contain caffeine. Although caffeine does help to trigger autophagy, and thus is included in the Hybrid Fast Latté, it is also a substance that the liver has to detoxify. It is up to you whether or not you choose to avoid caffeine completely. Caffeine also depresses melatonin, the sleep hormone, for up to 10 hours, so caffeinated drinks are generally best avoided after noon.

On our retreats my team provides ginger and turmeric tea, hibiscus tea and peppermint tea for participants to choose from. Ginger, turmeric and peppermint all aid digestion and calm the digestive tract. They work naturally to reduce gas and indigestion.

For those with particularly intransigent digestive systems we also give Blessed Herbs Digestive Stimulator capsules (see Resources), which combine aloe vera leaf, barberry root, cascara sagrada bark, Chinese rhubarb root, dandelion root, fennel seed, ginger root, liquorice root, meadowsweet (aerial parts) and peppermint leaf. Taking three capsules stimulates bowel movements. If this is a problem area for you, it would be wise to have a bottle at hand just in case you need this extra help.

The udiyanna bandha exercise to stimulate elimination

Also excellent in regard to relieving constipation is the classic yoga exercise udiyanna bandha. Whereas conventional exercise focuses on pulling in the belly to look slim and, in men, developing the six-pack look, it is also important for the abdominal area to be able to relax properly and to extend with the breath. While abdominal muscle-strengthening exercises such as sit-ups are good, you also need other kinds of abdominal exercise such as udiyanna bandha, which helps to stimulate digestion and massages the organs in the abdominal region. Here's how you do it:

Note Do not do this exercise if you are pregnant or menstruating or have stomach ulcers or a hernia.

Udiyanna bandha stomach exercise

1. Strand with your feet hip-width apart. Your shoulders, arms and hands are relaxed. Bend your knees and tilt your torso and head forward, bringing your hands to rest lightly on your thighs. Your head and spine are in a straight line. Avoid bending over too far. Check the buttock muscles remain relaxed.

2. Inhale through the nose then exhale sharply and empty your lungs completely. Contract your abdominal muscles fully to push as much air as possible out of your lungs. Then relax your abdominals. Keeping the lungs empty, alternately contract and relax the abdominal muscles in rapid succession ten times. Make each contraction as

deep as possible as you suck your belly button towards your spine. Keep the movements of the belly smooth and regular. The correct stance makes the contraction of the rectus abdominis muscle massage the viscera most effectively. You can feel the pull from the pubis bone up to the throat.

Summary

The 5-Day Diet provides:

- Foods that are high in soluble fibres.

- A glucomannan and vitamin C-rich drink to increase fibre and improve bowel elimination.

- Drinks, including teas, that ensure you achieve 2 litres of fluid a day, which helps the body to eliminate.

- Back-up herbs if constipation is a problem area for you.

Part 2

The Practical – How to Do it

Now you know how the diet works, this part will give you precise instructions so that you know exactly how to follow the 5-Day Diet and the sequence of drinks, foods, supplements and exercise. I'll also explain what you will need to stock up with to follow the diet and prepare the simple meals for each day.

Chapter 5

Getting Ready for Your 5-Day Diet

Plan ahead for when you want to follow the 5-Day Diet and read through this section to familiarise yourself with the way it will work for you. I'll first be explaining the role of the low-GL diet, as this is recommended as the diet to follow for a short period before you start the 5-Day Diet. You can use it to continue your weight-loss programme and, with minor adjustments, as a lifestyle choice for maintaining good health and your desired weight, as I will explain later in the book.

A few days before you're ready to start

I recommend preparing your body for the 5-Day Diet by following my low-GL slow-carb diet for a couple of days first. The diet is explained in full in Part 3. This is not a requirement, but if you go from a high-sugar diet straight into the five-day diet, it's going to be a bit of a shock to your system, so it's best to warm up first by getting used to a low- or no-sugar diet, eating slow carbs in the right amounts. In my original trial two people didn't do this preparation and it consequently took them a little longer to get into the zone.

Before you do a couple of days on my low-GL diet, it's important to understand the role of blood sugar in health as well as weight gain, and weight loss, as I explain in the box below.

The glycaemic load (GL) – and its role in weight

Keeping your blood sugar balanced is the concept at the heart of a low-GL diet, which I recommend you adopt as a weight-loss and lifestyle diet after you have completed the 5-Day Diet, because blood sugar highs and lows encourage weight gain, and energy dips, and are bad for overall health. You can achieve balanced blood sugar levels and sustainable weight loss if you follow a diet where foods high in what is known as the 'glycaemic load' (GL) are drastically reduced, and by controlling these foods you can maintain a healthy weight throughout life.

The GL is a unit of measurement that tells you exactly what a particular food will do to your blood sugar level. Foods with a high GL have a greater effect on your blood sugar, which isn't desirable. Foods with a low GL encourage the body to burn fat, which is what you're aiming for.

▶

When your blood sugar level increases, the hormone insulin is released into the bloodstream to remove the glucose (sugar). Some glucose goes to the brain and muscles, where it's used as an energy fuel, but any excess goes to the liver where it's turned into fat and stored, causing you to gain weight. Insulin is known as the fat-storing hormone.

The glycaemic load (GL) is based on the glycaemic index (GI). Put simply, the glycaemic index of a food tells you whether the carbohydrate in a food is fast- or slow-releasing (fast is bad, slow is good). What it doesn't tell you, though, is exactly *how much* of the food is carbohydrate. The glycaemic load, on the other hand, factors in both the *type* and the *amount* of carbohydrate in the food and consequently what that particular food in that amount will do to your blood sugar.

In a low-GL diet the carbs are restricted to enable the body to lose weight. During the 5-Day Diet the carbs will be even lower to encourage autophagy. You then move on to eating my low-GL slow-carb diet to maintain health. Although the 5-Day Diet focuses on the health benefits of autophagy, the diet also kick-starts weight loss and enables you to maintain a healthy weight, even later in life, when it can be more difficult. In Part 3 I explain how you can follow on from the 5-Day Diet by eating a low-GL diet to continue losing weight or with slightly more carbs to maintain your current weight and to keep your blood sugar levels even and healthy.

How to blend the diets

I recommend that you refer to Part 3 and eat in the way described there for at least two days before starting the 5-Day Diet, then make your last dinner low GL and eat it at 6.30pm, without a drink or dessert. This will give you an 18-hour carb fast before starting Day 1 with the Hybrid Fast Latté, which is essentially carb-free (I describe this drink later in this chapter). So your first carb-containing meal will be lunch at 12.30, giving you this 18-hour carb-free window. Following this plan will ensure that you get the most benefit from the five days that follow. I also recommend that you avoid alcohol for 48 hours before the diet as well as during the five days.

The 5-Day Diet overview

Before we get into the 'how to' of the 5-Day Diet it's worth taking an overview of what we are aiming to achieve so that you understand all the different components. Everything is designed to get you into ketosis fast and running on ketones as opposed to glucose. (Remember, your body can use fat to make ketones when glucose is not available.) This will then trigger the cellular self-repair process, autophagy, and optimise your ability to detoxify, by supporting the liver with key detox nutrients, and healthy elimination via the digestive tract.

From a nutritional point of view this diet is about precise engineering, much like getting a Formula 1 car to maximum performance. You don't *need* to know all the details, and you can skip to the next chapter to get started, if you like, but it's worth knowing the essential principles so that you don't veer from the path and inadvertently switch off autophagy.

These are the critical principles:

Low calorie The daily total of calories averages at 800. Much more than this might turn off autophagy.

Low carb and low GL The 5-Day Diet aims to deliver no more than 30g of carbohydrates a day. Lowering carbs is essential to lose weight on a low-carb diet. It is even more important to keep carbs very low on a ketogenic diet because the higher your blood sugar level goes the more insulin you make, and that says 'growth' and turns off both autophagy and ketosis. You'll learn, in Part 3, when you go on to a low-GL diet following the 5-Day Diet, that your allowance is 45–60 GLs a day; however, during the 5-Day Diet you mustn't eat more than 15 GLs a day, so everything is calculated to achieve this and, as you learn about the components (meals, snacks and drinks), I'll let you know how many GLs they contain. Read Part 3 if you want to understand the glycaemic load better. Fifteen GLs/30g is approximately 15 per cent of your total calories coming from carbs.

Low protein Your protein intake is limited to 25g. This is roughly half what you need on a regular basis, but it is fine for five days. Protein, and especially meat and dairy protein, sends a growth signal to your body, which switches off autophagy. Twenty-five grams of protein is about 15 per cent of your total calories.

High fat and ketogenic Percentagewise, the 5-Day Diet is high fat because about 70 per cent of your calories will come from fat, but actually it'll only be about 60g a day because you'll be eating low calories overall. Fat is satiating. You'll also be eating the kind of fats the body easily converts into ketones for energy.

An 18-hour carb fast You are going to start each day with a Hybrid Fast Latté, which is virtually carb-free, having eaten dinner the night before at 6 or 7pm, then you will have a very low-carb snack mid-morning, and lunch at noon or 1pm. This means that you will effectively start each day with an 18-hour carb fast. You'll have a more substantial mid-afternoon snack, then dinner with a treat before bed.

High in autophagy triggers and detox nutrients The foods, drinks and supplements are all designed to encourage auto-phagy, and support detoxification, which will happen as you break down body fat. The exact sequence of the supplements and the drinks is important to follow. They'll also deliver a substantial amount of the super-soluble fibre glucomannan, and vitamin C, both of which help healthy elimination, which can be an issue on a low-calorie and high-fat diet, as we saw in Chapter 4.

It's very important not to adapt the diet without considering all these principles. If you increase the protein, or the calories or the carbs, that can switch off autophagy and negate the benefit of the 5-Day Diet.

Each day on the 5-Day Diet

You will have the following on each of the five days:

- The Hybrid Fast Latté in the morning (explained opposite).

- A drink made with glucomannan and vitamin C, which you will take three times a day, throughout the day (explained on page 62).

- A specific morning snack that you buy, ready-made (there is also a home-made option, which I explain later in this section).

- A mid-afternoon Get Up & Go shake (explained on page 64) or you can repeat the morning snack.

- Lunches and dinners that you make, as discussed later.

- Supplements – these are a vital part of the 5-Day Diet because they help to trigger autophagy, as explained on pages 29–32. In Chapter 8 I'll let you know what to buy and when to take them during the five days.

The next chapter lays out in detail the daily routine for you to follow, but before we get into this you need to know how to make the Hybrid Fast Latté, the glucomannan and vitamin C drink, and the Get Up & Go shake, which is your best option for an afternoon snack.

Your morning routine and the Hybrid Fast Latté

As we have seen, a fast way to trigger autophagy and ketosis is an 18-hour carb fast. This means having dinner at 6 or 7pm and lunch at noon or 1pm. This should be your routine for each of the five days. At noon on the sixth day, you start on the low-GL lifestyle diet if you wish to (explained in Part 3).

On the diet days you will, no doubt, wake up hungry, but

even though your first meal is not until noon or 1pm, you do not need to go without consuming anything at all. Your first 'meal' of the day is my fasting version of the Hybrid Latté, each of the ingredients of which has an important role to play in the diet. They are:

Carb-free almond milk It's very important to buy a brand that says 'zero carbs'. Check the nutritional ingredients on the back of the carton for the carbohydrate content, which must say 0. Alpro makes an unsweetened roasted or unroasted almond milk, for example.

Coffee helps to kick-start ketosis and autophagy, but it's OK to use decaf if you prefer, or to have no coffee at all.

Almond butter Of all the nuts, almonds are the best choice because they are very low in carbs. A level tablespoon, or a heaped dessertspoon, will give you only about 2g of carbs, plenty of healthy fats and some protein. This amount of carbs is not enough to take you out of ketosis.

C8 oil As we saw in Chapter 1, the fat or oil from which the body can directly make ketones in the liver, thereby switching on ketosis, is caprylic acid triglyceride or C8 oil. Ketofast is one brand of 99 per cent C8 oil that is derived from pure coconut oil, not palm oil. (It doesn't matter which brand you buy as long as it's pure C8 oil, and I prefer coconut-oil derived C8 for environmental reasons.) Brain cells prefer this fuel to glucose, so you'll find that your mind becomes focused after the Hybrid Latté; however, please bear in mind that it takes a few days for your body to adapt to it, and, if you start with too high an amount, you can experience diarrhoea or stomach cramps. This will resolve as your body gets used to this new source of fuel. Unlike other fats, C8 oil goes straight to the liver via the portal vein (a vein connecting the stomach and intestines to the liver), and thus it does not require all the digestion that other fats need.

The ketones then enter the blood and are taken up as an energy source by the cells' mitochondria (the energy factories). The optimal amount to take is 2 to 3 tablespoons a day, but it's wise to start with 2 to 3 *teaspoons* a day. On Day 1, therefore, just put one teaspoon in your Hybrid Latté. If you're OK with this, use a dessertspoon (two teaspoons) on Day 2 and a tablespoon (three teaspoons) on Day 3, then keep going with this amount on the subsequent days.

Cacao powder The health benefits of cacao hinge on its high levels of flavonoids, mainly epicatechins and catechins. These are powerful polyphenols, acting as antioxidants and helping to maintain a healthy cardiovascular system. It also contains a mild stimulant, theobromine, and has a lovely taste. Cacao also helps to trigger autophagy.

Cinnamon Of all the spices, cinnamon is my favourite. It helps to stabilise blood sugar and is therefore especially good for those with blood sugar problems. It also helps to trigger autophagy.

The recipe for the Hybrid Fast Latté

120ml no-carb almond milk (unsweetened)
120ml filtered coffee (less caffeine, more antioxidants)
1 level tbsp (16g) almond butter
1–3 tsp C8 oil (such as Ketofast)
½ rounded tsp cacao powder
⅓ tsp cinnamon

Blend all the ingredients in a blender or NutriBullet. If you'd like it hot (it will be warm from the coffee), heat it up in a saucepan. If you like it cold, as in an iced latté, pour it over some ice cubes.

You'll be having a mid-morning snack, ideally two hours after your Hybrid Fast Latté and two hours before your lunch; for example, if you had your Hybrid Fast Latté at 8.30am you'd have your snack around 10.30am and your lunch at 12.30pm.

Your Carboslow and ImmuneC drink

In addition to the Hybrid Fast Latté you'll also fill up a 500ml water container with the combo of glucomannan fibre and vitamin C. Carboslow glucomannan and ImmuneC powder are two specific products that are sugar-free and taste good, so that's what we use on our retreats. If you can't get these, make sure that both the glucomannan powder and vitamin C powder you choose are sugar-free. These are available in health-food shops. You'll need a 500ml, transparent, ideally wide-lidded container or water bottle. You can use a 1-litre bottle and fill it up halfway (or make up 1.5 litres of water with the mixture and drink a third of this during the morning, afternoon and evening). You should drink your 500ml of mixture throughout the morning, for example, so that it is empty by lunchtime, and repeat with the refills for the rest of the day. This will help to fill you up.

The recipe for the Carboslow and ImmuneC drink

500ml water, filtered or bottled if possible

½ tsp (2.5g), or 1 scoop using the scoop provided,
Carboslow glucomannan fibre
level ½ tsp ImmuneC High Potency powder or pure
ascorbic acid*

Pour the water into your transparent drinking bottle. Add the glucomannan and ImmuneC powder. Put on the top and shake well. Shake the bottle several times during the first 10 minutes of making the mixture so that the fibre completely dissolves in the water.

* Although you can use pure ascorbic acid powder, ImmuneC powder has certain berry extracts that help it to taste sweet, rather than tart, but is sugar-free, as well being high in minerals such as magnesium. If you do use any other vitamin C powder it must be sugar-free with zero carbs.

Mid-morning snacks

During mid morning you have one of two snacks – seaweed crispies or kale crackers – with five olives, ideally pitted Kalamata olives. Both kale and seaweed [1] promote autophagy. We use Clearspring SeaVeg Crispies made from toasted nori seaweed on our retreats. A pack contains 28 calories and 1.7g of carbs, which is less than 1 GL. Online suppliers are given in the Resources if you can't find these in your health-food shop. If you find alternatives, make sure that they don't contain more calories or carbs.

The kale crackers are home-made. If you opt for these, your snack allowance is three kale crackers, plus five olives. The recipe is given on page 78.

Your mid-afternoon snack

For your mid-afternoon snack, roughly between lunch and dinner, you can repeat your mid-morning snacks; however, there is a more filling option, which also gives you more gluco-mannan fibre and is compliant with the diet's requirement of low calorie and low GL. You can make a shake using the shake powder, Get Up & Go with Carboslow, plus no-carb almond milk and berries. Get Up & Go with Carboslow is an incredibly low-GL shake, which many people have for breakfast. It is made from whole foods: apple powder for carbs, a protein combo from quinoa, soya and rice protein, ground almonds and seeds, cinnamon and oat fibre, as well as glucomannan fibre. Together with the fibre in Carboslow you'll achieve the ideal intake, both for regular bowels and making you feel fuller, hence reducing your appetite so that you're not hungry. Get Up & Go with Carboslow also contains many vitamins and minerals which, together with those recommended in Chapter 6, brings you to the ideal intake to both trigger autophagy and help detoxification. Get Up & Go with Carboslow, for the usual 30g serving (a heaped tablespoon), has an exceptionally low GL of 4; however, you'll be having a half portion, 15g, which is only 2 GLs. With carb-free milk, and a handful of berries, this is about 2.5 GLs. It will look like a small glass (or half a large glass) of a thickish milkshake.

This will be your mid-afternoon snack. If, for example, you had lunch at 1pm and plan to have dinner at 7pm, have this snack at 4pm.

The recipe for the Get Up & Go with Carboslow Shake

1 heaped dessertspoon (2 heaped tsp) (15g) Get Up & Go
with Carboslow powder
150ml (1 small glass) no-carb almond milk
a small handful of frozen berries (such as 12 blueberries or
6 strawberries)

Put the Get Up & Go powder, almond milk and frozen berries
in a blender or food processor and blend until smooth or to your
preferred consistency. Serve.

An after-dinner treat

After dinner there's a small treat for you. You can have either
three Chocolate Almonds, which you can make yourself (see
the recipe on page 83), or a Nibble Protein Bite: Lemon with
Coconut (see Resources). These are 21 calories, 2g of carbs, so
less than 1 GL.

Breaking your fast

On Day 6 you will not want to be eating too much as your
stomach will have shrunk, therefore it's good to have smaller
proportions but with enough to fill you up, and also to not
go too heavy on meat and dairy products, which you've
been avoiding.

Breakfast on Day 6

For breakfast I recommend you have either:

A small bowl of oats with chia seeds or chopped almonds and berries, perhaps with oat or almond milk.

Or

One or two scrambled eggs on a piece of rye bread or two oatcakes.

Or

A Get up & Go shake, blended with berries and milk (this is the original version of Get Up & Go, without the Carboslow, which has a slightly higher GL but still below 10 GLs for a full serving with dairy milk, almond or oat milk).

If you prefer to start with a Hybrid Latté and make your first meal more of a brunch, that's fine too. If you do this you could have the eggs with some smoked salmon and avocado.

Lunch on Day 6

A very good and easy-to-make soup for lunch is my Chestnut and Butter Bean Soup (see page 164). Chestnuts have the lowest fat content of all nuts and a pleasantly sweet flavour that goes well with the creamy texture of the blended butter beans. This is very filling and cooks quickly with minimal effort.

Dinner on Day 6 and onward

Thereafter, pick any of the low-GL recipes or meals in Chapter 12. I recommend that you stay off alcohol for at least 24, if not 48, hours after finishing the five days.

The 5-Day Diet Daily Routine – Day by Day

In this chapter I set out your schedule of what to eat and drink at different times of the day during your 5-Day Diet and how to prepare and maintain your body with exercise. In Chapter 7 you will find a shopping list to help you get everything organised in advance. The recipes for all the meals listed below are also included in Chapter 7. Recipes for the Latte, the glucomannan drink and the Get Up & Go shake are in Chapter 6.

The timings given in the schedules are a guide only, based on what my team and I do during our Hybrid Fast Detox Retreats (see Resources). If you're an owl by nature, you can always move everything forward, but the gaps between meals are important, as is the 18-hour carb fast between dinner and lunch the next day. I recommend exercising at 8.30am, but if you don't like to exercise so early, choose a time that suits you before lunch or before dinner, but not after a meal.

Exercise – how much should you take?

Your body has two phases: growth and repair. During the 5-Day Diet your body is in the *repair* phase, therefore you don't want to be working to grow muscles, which is what strength or resistance training does. Too much resistance-type exercise will turn autophagy off.

If you do absolutely no exercise, however, your body, starved of glucose, will turn to protein, which is found in the muscles, and will break it down to convert into glucose. That is why people on total fasts lose muscle mass, which is the last thing you want, especially if you are older. For this reason the 5-Day Diet includes some protein, but not too much to switch off autophagy.

In addition, you will benefit from doing a small amount of cardio or aerobic exercise every day during the diet. If, for example, you cycle, swim or jog for 15 minutes, or a maximum of 30 minutes walking if you are fit, you are unlikely to switch off autophagy. Also, this exercise tells your muscles that they're still needed, thus protecting against loss of muscle mass. You could also get away with a short session of resistance training, but don't overdo it. These five days are not about building muscle; they are about repair, so take it easy.

You should be exercising at a level where you are breathing more heavily but still able to talk. If you have to stop because you're puffed out, you're going too fast. If you are monitoring your pulse, this should increase to above 100 beats a minute, but below 120 beats per minute, within 5 minutes of exercising.

The best time to do your aerobic exercise is before, not after, a meal. Evolutionarily, this makes sense: we'd hunt or gather, then eat – not the other way around. This could be on rising, before your Hybrid Latté, or before lunch. On my retreats we have two circuits, one flatter for the less fit and one hillier for the more fit, each taking about 15 minutes to complete. The very fit people do this twice. You might have a similar route near you: around the block or local park, for example. It is best to decide on your route and then do this every day. But remember not to push yourself too hard.

A recommended exercise routine

In my *Burn Fat Fast* book, personal trainer and former gladiator (Zodiac) Kate Staples provides an excellent routine, which comprises an eight-minute strengthening and resistance workout every other day and a 30-minute cardio workout three times a week. A 45-minute brisk walk or cycle ride twice a week would also suffice. The eight-minute strengthening workout is composed of four exercises that vary in difficulty depending on whether you are a beginner, intermediate or advanced (for example, a full press-up is advanced level), with each exercise done twice for one minute. All the exercises can be done anywhere without any specialist equipment, although, as you advance, it might be worth investing in some hand weights, to take the place of water bottles. To find out more, see www.hybriddiet.co.uk/exercise.

You could halve this – for example a four-minute strength and resistance workout and a 15-minute cardio workout every other day. The strength and resistance exercises are based on repeating each exercise twice, so you'd be just doing them once.

Prepare for the diet by exercising the day before

On the day before you start the 5-Day Diet, I strongly recommend that you have an extensive cardio or aerobic exercise session – ideally before a meal. The reason for this is that first thing in the morning, for example, before you've had a carb-loaded breakfast, your blood glucose level is quite low. As you exercise you'll burn through your blood glucose and your body will start to break down stores of glucose, held as glycogen, in your muscles and liver. The more you deplete glycogen stores the faster you are going to go into ketosis, switching to burning ketones instead of glucose.

What this means depends very much on your level of fitness, but you should be pushing yourself to the limit with a long walk, ideally with some hills, or cycle, jog or swim, or take a one-hour exercise class. For most people, glycogen stores are depleted with 60–90 minutes of moderate-intensity exercise. Twelve to 18 hours fasting also uses this up, so with dinner at 7pm on the day before you start, then a Hybrid Fast Latté on the morning of Day 1, and with lunch at 1pm, you should be in ketosis, switching from burning carbs to burning fat.

Now that you understand the basic principles of exercise during this time, overleaf you will find your schedule for exercise and what to eat and take as supplements for the five days of the diet.

Day 1

8am	Cardio exercise; for example, 15 minutes of brisk walking.
8.30am	Hybrid Fast Latté (see page 61 for recipe). Supplements: 1 × GL Support; 1 strip of Hybrid Pack or equivalent (see Chapter 8). Drink: 500ml container of Carboslow and ImmuneC drink (page 63). Drink it by lunchtime.
10.15am	Snack – Seaweed Crispies (5g pack) (see Resources) or Kale Crackers (page 78) and 5 pitted Kalamata olives.
12.30pm	Lunch – Scrambled Egg and Asparagus (page 79) served with kimchi (see Resources). Supplements: 1 × GL Support. Drink: 500ml Carboslow and ImmuneC (as above). Drink it by dinnertime.
3pm	Snack – Get Up & Go with Carboslow (2.5g) shake (page 65) or repeat your morning snack.
6.30pm	Dinner – Mushroom Soup (page 80). Supplements: 1 × GL Support. Drink: 500ml Carboslow and ImmuneC (as above). Drink it by the morning. Dessert: Nibble one Protein Bite: Lemon with Coconut (see Resources).
8pm or before bed	Hot bath with Epsom salts (see box on page 96).

Day 2

8am   Cardio exercise, as Day 1.

8.30am   Hybrid Fast Latté.
                Supplements: 1 × GL Support; 1 strip of Hybrid
                Pack or equivalent.
                Drink: 500ml container of Carboslow and
                ImmuneC. Drink it by lunchtime.

10.15am   Snack – Seaweed Crispies (5g pack) (see
                Resources) and 5 pitted Kalamata olives.

12.30pm   Lunch – Guacamole (see page 81 for recipe),
                served with kimchi.
                Supplements: 1 × GL Support.
                Drink: Reload your 500ml container with
                Carboslow and ImmuneC drink. Drink it by
                dinnertime.

3pm   Snack – Get Up & Go with Carboslow shake,
                or repeat your morning snack.

6.30pm   Dinner – Watercress, Leek and Coconut Soup
                (page 82) served with Kale Crackers (page 78).
                Supplements: 1 × GL Support.
                Drink: 500ml Carboslow and ImmuneC (as
                above). Drink it by the morning.
                Dessert: 3 Dark Chocolate Almonds (page 83).

8pm or before   Hot bath with Epsom salts.
bed

Day 3

8am	Cardio exercise, as Day 1.
8.30am	Hybrid Fast Latté. Supplements: 1 × GL Support; 1 strip of Hybrid Pack or equivalent. Drink: 500ml container of Carboslow and ImmuneC drink. Drink it by lunchtime.
10.15am	Snack – Seaweed crispies (5g pack) and 5 pitted Kalamata olives.
12.30pm	Lunch – Marinated Salmon with Spinach and Kale (see page 84 for recipe) Supplements: 1 × GL Support. Drink: Reload your 500ml container with Carboslow and ImmuneC drink. Drink it by dinnertime.
3pm	Snack – Get Up & Go with Carboslow shake, or repeat your morning snack.
6.30pm	Dinner – Roasted Tomato and Basil Soup (page 85) served with Kale Crackers (page 78). Supplements: 1 × GL Support. Drink: 500ml Carboslow and ImmuneC (as above). Drink it by the morning. Dessert: Nibble one Protein Bite: Lemon with Coconut.
8pm or before bed	Hot bath with Epsom salts.

Day 4

8am	Cardio exercise, as Day 1.
8.30am	Hybrid Fast Latté. Supplements: 1 × GL Support; 1 strip of Hybrid Pack or equivalent. Drink: 500ml container of Carboslow and ImmuneC drink. Drink it by lunchtime.
10.15am	Snack – Seaweed Crispies (5g pack) and 5 pitted Kalamata olives.
12.30pm	Lunch – Smoked Tofu, Walnut and Artichoke Salad (see page 85 for recipe), served with kimchi. Supplements: 1 × GL Support. Drink: Reload your 500ml container with Carboslow and ImmuneC drink. Drink it by dinnertime.
3pm	Snack – Get Up & Go with Carboslow shake, or repeat your morning snack.
6.30pm	Dinner – Cauliflower and Broccoli Soup (page 86). Supplements: 1 × GL Support. Drink: 500ml Carboslow and ImmuneC (as above). Drink it by the morning. Dessert: 3 Dark Chocolate Almonds.
8pm or before bed	Hot bath with Epsom salts.

Day 5

8am   Cardio exercise, as Day 1.

8.30am   Hybrid Fast Latté.
Supplements: 1 × GL Support; 1 strip of Hybrid Pack or equivalent.
Drink: 500ml container of Carboslow and ImmuneC drink. Drink it by lunchtime.

10.15am   Snack – Seaweed Crispies (5g pack) and 5 pitted Kalamata olives.

12.30pm   Lunch – Sardine Salad (see page 87 for recipe), served with kimchi.
Supplements: 1 × GL Support.
Drink: Reload your 500ml container with Carboslow and ImmuneC drink. Drink it by dinnertime.

3pm   Snack – Get Up & Go with Carboslow shake, or repeat your morning snack.

6.30pm   Dinner – Patrick's Primordial Soup (page 88).
Supplements: 1 × GL Support.
Drink: 500ml Carboslow and ImmuneC (as above). Drink it by the morning.
Dessert: Nibble one Protein Bite: Lemon with Coconut.

8pm or before bed   Hot bath with Epsom salts.

Note The lunches and soups for dinner are interchangeable, so, if you prefer one to another, you can have it more than once. At its simplest, you could choose the one you like best and make enough for the five days; however, variation is more satisfying, hence you have five options to choose from, both for lunch and dinner. I have also included in each recipe ingredients that will help to trigger autophagy.

Chapter 7

The Recipes and Shopping Lists

I n this chapter you will find the recipes for the meals given in the previous chapter. The Latté, Carboslow and ImmuneC drink and Get Up & Go with Carboslow shake can be found in Chapter 5, where you will also find details of my suggested sea-weed crispies or protein nibbles. If you can't find these, or want to make your your own snack, substitute Kale Crackers, as follows:

Kale Crackers

Makes 30 crackers
1 large handful kale, ribs removed, chopped in the food processor to make into a pulp
2 garlic cloves, crushed
1 tbsp very finely chopped rosemary
170g ground flax

40g chia seeds
40g sesame seeds
1 tbsp fresh lemon juice
1 tbsp olive oil
salt to taste

1. Preheat the oven to 100°C (80°C fan oven) Gas ¼.

2. Place all the ingredients in a large glass bowl and mix
    with your hands until they form a ball. Place the ball
    between two sheets of parchment and roll out with a
    rolling pin as thin as possible, without breaking any of
    the edges.

3. Put the rolled out dough on a baking sheet and use a
    pizza cutter to score the dough into approximately 30
    crackers. Bake for about 45 minutes and then turn. Bake
    for another 45 minutes or until crisp on both sides. Allow
    to cool then break into crackers.

Day 1

Scrambled Egg and Asparagus

Serves 1
1 large egg
4 asparagus spears (64g)
100g kimchi, to serve

Dressing:
1 tsp tahini
1 tsp olive oil

ground black pepper
a squeeze of lemon juice

1. Put the dressing ingredients in a small bowl and mix well together.

2. Put the egg in a bowl and add a splash of water, then whisk gently.

3. Bring a pan of water to the boil and add the asparagus. Cook for 3–6 minutes, until al dente or according to preference, then drain.

4. While the asparagus is cooking, add the egg mixture to a cold pan over a medium–low heat and cook, stirring with a wooden spoon, until scrambled to your preferred consistency.

5. Serve the asparagus drizzled with the dressing, with the egg and the kimchi.

Mushroom Soup

Serves 1
1 tsp olive oil
2 tsp finely chopped shallots
1 garlic clove, crushed
75g mushrooms, cut into quarters
2 tsp almond flour
240ml vegetable bouillon or stock
a pinch of freshly grated nutmeg
a pinch of finely chopped fresh coriander
ground black pepper
3 Kale Crackers, to serve

1. Heat the oil in a saucepan over a medium heat and add the shallots and garlic. Cook for 5 minutes or until tender.

2. Add the mushrooms and cook, stirring, until lightly browned.

3. Stir in the almond flour until the mushrooms and onions are coated. Add the stock in small amounts, stirring to ensure that the flour is absorbed and there are no lumps.

4. Add the nutmeg and coriander, and bring to the boil. Reduce the heat and simmer gently until the soup thickens, stirring occasionally.

5. Purée using a blender or food processor to your desired consistency and add black pepper to taste. Serve with the kale crackers.

Day 2

Guacamole

Serves 1
¼ small red onion, very finely chopped
½ small avocado
lime juice, to taste
1 tsp apple cider vinegar
1 tsp very finely chopped coriander
1 small roasted garlic clove (optional) (see tip)
100g kimchi and 3 Kale Crackers, to serve

1. Put the onion in a bowl and add the garlic, if using.

2. Remove the avocado pit and scoop out the flesh using a tablespoon. Add it to the bowl and squeeze over a little lime juice to stop it from going brown. Mash using a fork.

3. Add the apple cider vinegar and coriander, and mix to your preferred consistency. If you prefer a smoother guacamole, use a hand blender. Serve with the kimchi and kale crackers.

Tip Crushed fresh garlic can be used, but roasted will give it a milder, sweeter flavour.

Watercress, Leek and Coconut Soup

Serves 1
1 tsp olive oil
½ onion, chopped
1 small garlic clove, crushed
½ leek, white part only, finely sliced
40g watercress, plus extra to serve
75ml coconut milk
185ml vegetable bouillon or stock
salt and ground black pepper
3 Kale Crackers, to serve

1. Heat the oil in a saucepan over a medium heat and cook the onion and garlic for 3–4 minutes until softened.

2. Add the leek, watercress, coconut milk and stock, then bring to the boil. Reduce the heat to low, then cover and simmer for 5–10 minutes until the leeks are tender.

3. Remove from the heat and allow to cool slightly, then purée using a blender or food processor until smooth.

Add salt to taste, reheat if necessary, then grind over black pepper, garnish with extra watercress and serve with kale crackers.

Dark Chocolate Almonds

If you decide to make a smaller quantity than the recipe below, note that half a square of chocolate will cover three almonds. Portion size: 3 almonds

100g bar dark 85 per cent cocoa solids chocolate, such as Lindt 85 per cent dark chocolate, broken into pieces
1 tsp coconut oil
a sprinkle of sea salt or chilli powder
2 × 300g packs almonds (not roasted, sweetened or salted)

1. Line a baking tray with baking parchment. Melt the chocolate in a heatproof bowl over a pan of gently simmering water, making sure that the base of the bowl doesn't touch the water. Stir in the coconut oil and add a sprinkle of sea salt or chilli powder.

2. Once the chocolate has melted, add the nuts in batches, making sure they are well coated.

3. Put the nuts on the prepared baking tray and chill in the refrigerator for a few hours or overnight until set. Store in an airtight container.

Day 3

Marinated Salmon with Spinach and Kale

Serves 1
25g piece of salmon steak
½ tsp coconut oil
100g kale
100g spinach
100g of kimchi, to serve

Marinade:

juice of ¼ lemon
a pinch of ground cumin
a pinch of ground coriander
¼ tsp Dijon mustard

1. Preheat the oven to 180°C (160°C fan oven) Gas 4. Mix
    the marinade ingredients together in a small bowl and
    coat the salmon in the mixture. Put the salmon on a
    piece of baking paper or foil and splash over a little
    water, then wrap the salmon in the paper and put it on a
    baking tray. Cook in the oven for 10 minutes.

2. While the salmon is cooking, heat the oil in a saucepan
    over a medium heat and cook the kale for 5 minutes,
    then add the spinach and cook until creamy. Serve the
    salmon and green vegetables with the kimchi.

Tip Garlic, freshly grated nutmeg or cayenne pepper can
be added to the kale and spinach mix for added flavour,
if you like.

Roasted Tomato and Basil Soup

Serves 1
2 large tomatoes, cut in half
1 garlic clove, chopped
¼ onion, cut in half
125ml vegetable bouillon or stock
2 tsp finely chopped basil
1 tsp olive oil
3 Kale Crackers

1. Preheat the oven to 200°C (180°C fan oven) Gas 6. Put the tomatoes cut-side up in a roasting tin. Add the garlic and onion, and drizzle with olive oil.

2. Season and roast for 15–20 minutes until the tomatoes are slightly browned but not burnt. Remove from the oven and put into a saucepan over a medium heat.

3. Add the stock and bring to the boil. Add the basil, then reduce the heat and simmer for 10 minutes. Purée using a blender or food processor. Serve with the kale crackers.

Day 4

Smoked Tofu, Walnut and Artichoke Salad

Serves 1
1 packet of baby leaf and rocket salad
40g smoked tofu, cut into cubes
4 artichoke hearts marinated in brine

2 tbsp chopped walnuts
100g kimchi, to serve

Dressing:

1 tsp tahini
1 tsp olive oil
juice of ½ lemon
ground black pepper

1. Put the dressing ingredients in a small bowl and mix together.

2. Put the leaf salad in a small serving bowl and add the tofu, artichokes and walnuts. Pour over the dressing and serve with the kimchi.

Tip Try baking the tofu on a baking sheet in an oven preheated to 200°C (180°C fan oven) Gas 6 for 10–15 minutes to make crunchy croutons for added texture.

Cauliflower and Broccoli Soup

Serves 1
¼ head of cauliflower, evenly chopped into small pieces
½ crown of broccoli, evenly chopped into small pieces
16g hemp seeds
½ tbsp garlic olive oil
240ml vegetable bouillon or stock, plus extra if needed
16g nutritional yeast (see Resources), or to taste
¼ tsp garlic powder
a pinch of dried thyme
salt and ground black pepper

1. Put the cauliflower and broccoli in a pan of boiling water and cook for 5 minutes or until tender.

2. Meanwhile, blend the hemp seeds, 115ml water and the garlic olive oil in a blender or mini food processor for 1 minute or until smooth.

3. Drain the cauliflower and broccoli in a colander and put it back into the pan. Add the creamy garlic mixture and the vegetable stock, and blend until smooth.

4. Add the nutritional yeast, garlic powder and dried thyme to the veg mixture and stir. You might need to add more stock to the mixture, as the hemp seeds will absorb a lot of water.

5. Season to taste. Add more nutritional yeast for more of a 'cheesy' flavour if you like.

For the almond recipe for dessert, see Day 2, page 83.

Day 5

Sardine Salad

Serves 1
½ can sardines
¼ small red onion, roughly chopped
a pinch of finely chopped coriander
a pinch of finely chopped flat leaf parsley
juice of ¼ lemon
4 capers
½ tbsp apple cider vinegar

1 tbsp olive oil
salt and ground black pepper
rocket and mixed baby leaf salad, 100g portion of kimchi, and
3 Kale Crackers, to serve

Put all the ingredients in a blender or food processer and blend
together. Serve with the leaf salad, kimchi and kale crackers.

Patrick's Primordial Soup

Serves 1
1 tsp olive oil
¼ red onion, roughly chopped
1 small garlic clove, crushed
1 carrot, chopped
½ tsp fresh root ginger, peeled and grated
a pinch of ground turmeric
1 tsp bouillon powder
¼ red pepper, deseeded and roughly chopped
2½ tbsp coconut milk

1. Heat the oil in a saucepan over a medium heat and cook
    the onion and garlic for 3–4 minutes until softened.

2. Add the carrot, ginger, turmeric and bouillon powder.
    Add boiling water to just cover and bring to the boil.
    Reduce the heat, cover and simmer for 10 minutes or until
    the carrot is soft.

3. Add the red pepper and coconut milk, reheat if needed,
    then purée using a blender or food processor until smooth
    and thick. Serve.

Your shopping lists

Here is your food shopping list followed by a list of the supplements and the quantities you will need to buy before you start the 5-Day Diet. Some of the supplements are sold in larger amounts than you will require for the five days, but you can use them in the future if you repeat the diet or share them if you have a friend who wants to join you on the diet.

Food

All the foods listed are best sourced as organic, if you can, as you are detoxifying your body and it is therefore preferable to avoid pesticide and herbicide residues.

Fresh herbs and flavourings:

2 packs fresh coriander   a small piece of fresh ginger
1 pack fresh basil   1 pack flat leaf parsley
1 garlic bulb   1 pack fresh rosemary

Vegetables and salads:

asparagus (you will   1 leek
need 4 spears)   75g mushrooms
1 small avocado   2 red onions
2 packs baby leaf and   1 red pepper
rocket salad   4 shallots
½ head of broccoli   100g spinach
¼ cauliflower   2 large tomatoes
1 carrot   40g watercress
small bag kale

Fruit:

3 lemons

1 lime

Fresh foods:

½ dozen eggs

1 pack smoked tofu

25g piece salmon steak

Tins and jars:

1 tin coconut milk

1 tin sardines in spring water

1 small jar capers

artichoke hearts marinated
in brine, tinned or in a jar

1 jar pitted Kalamata olives

tahini (H)

coconut oil

Dijon mustard

Meridian smooth almond
butter (H, this also comes in
a 1kg tub, see Resources)

Dried herbs and spices:

black pepper

ground cinnamon

ground coriander

ground cumin

whole nutmeg

dried thyme

ground turmeric

Grocery, general:

3 litres no-carb almond milk

1 small pack almond flour (H)

2 packs whole almonds, 300g

1 small pot cacao powder (H)

1 bar dark chocolate, 85 per
cent cocoa solids

1 pack ground coffee/decaf

hemp seeds (H)

ground flax seed

chia seeds

sesame seeds

1 small bottle garlic olive oil

Marigold vegetable
bouillon powder

nutritional yeast (H, see
Resources)

olive oil

1 small bag of
chopped walnuts

Crisps and snacks:

2 jars Eaten Alive Classic
Mild Kimchi (H)
1 pack Nibble Protein Bites:
Lemon with Coconut (H)

Organic Seaweed
Crispies (H)

(H) These foods are more likely to be found in a health-food store. In case you can't find any of the above essentials there, the Resources section gives you links to the direct suppliers. Most health-food stores can get these more specialist foods if you ask them to, however.

Supplements

1 bottle Ketofast, which contains 33 servings (33 tablespoons). You need a maximum of 15 but will start with teaspoons not tablespoons. This will give you enough for three 5-Day Diet cycles, although you may wish to continue having in Hybrid Lattés or on its own.

1 × Hybrid Pack (28 strips). You need 5 strips. This will give you enough for five 5-Day Diet cycles, although you can continue to take these. (For alternatives, see page 94.)

1 × GL Support with Carnitine (90 pills). You need 15 pills. This will give you enough for six 5-Day Diet cycles, but you can keep taking these. (For alternatives, see page 95.)

1 tub of Get Up & Go with Carboslow (10 × 30g servings). You need 5 × 15g servings = 75g. This will give you enough for four 5-Day Diet cycles but you can continue to have a 30g portion as breakfast during the follow-on low-GL phase.

1 tub of Carboslow (200g). You need 7.5g × 5 servings = 37.5g. This will give you enough for five 5-Day Diet cycles. Alternatively, any glucomannan fibre in powder or capsules will suffice as long as it is not sweetened.

1 tub of ImmuneC High Strength powder (200g). You need 3g × 5 servings = 15g. This will give you enough for several 5-Day Diet sequences, and is great immune support in cold season. If difficult to find, any pure vitamin C powder, without added sugar, will suffice.

You can buy a '5-Day Diet' Combo, which provides enough to complete at least three 5-Day Diets (see Resources); however, I advise that you continue with these supplements during the low-carb lifestyle phase that you can follow after the diet, especially if you wish to lose weight.

You can also find alternatives for the Hybrid Pack and GL Support, see 'Alternative supplement options' on pages 94 and 95.

Chapter 8

Support Supplements

The support supplements I recommend during the 5-Day Diet include all those nutrients discussed in Part 1 that will support switching your metabolism from using glucose to ketones, thereby helping the body to burn fat and supporting the liver's ability to detoxify the toxins that are released as you do so.

In practical terms, the easiest way to achieve this is by taking, daily:

- 1 strip of the Hybrid Pack (this provides vitamin C, multivitamins and minerals, AGE antioxidants, and DHA-rich omega-3 fish oil). This is best taken with your Hybrid Fast Latté in the morning as described in Chapter 6.

- 3 × GL Support, which provides three vital metabolic nutrients – chromium, garcinia cambogia (a natural source of HCA), and carnitine. Take one with each meal, starting with your Hybrid Fast Latté in the morning.

In addition to these you'll be taking autophagy-friendly nutrients to get the full benefit of the diet, as well as nutrients that help to support healthy metabolism and detoxification, in both your Carboslow and ImmuneC drink and the mid-afternoon Get Up & Go snack, plus, of course, the super-healthy foods.

Collectively these provide:

Antioxidants, including alpha-lipoic acid, CoQ10 and resveratrol

B vitamins

Carnitine

Chromium

Glucomannan fibre (see Chapter 4)

HCA

Omega-3 fish oil rich in DHA

Vitamin C with berry extracts and ginger

Zinc, magnesium (plus other minerals)

Alternative supplement options

The Hybrid Pack is a daily strip containing a high-strength multivitamin and mineral, rich in: magnesium (155mg); 900mg of vitamin C with zinc (16mg); omega-3 and 6 fats providing 574mg of EPA and DHA; and an antioxidant supplement including alpha-lipoic acid, CoQ10, resveratrol and glutathione. If you prefer to use other products, make sure you include those four supplements.

GL Support is a combination of garcinia cambogia, providing HCA (2,250mg), chromium (225µg) and carnitine (100mg) in three tablets. These are the daily amounts of these key auto-phagy trigger nutrients you are shooting for. You will find plenty of choice for these nutrients individually in health food stores but not in combination.

Supplements to support the metabolism

To turn any food, be it protein, carbs or fat, into energy requires nutrients. In the diagram below you can see the key players, all of which I recommend you take in optimal amounts during the 5-Day Diet because they will help to optimise your ability to make energy within the mitochondria – the energy factories in cells.

Co-factor nutrients for making energy

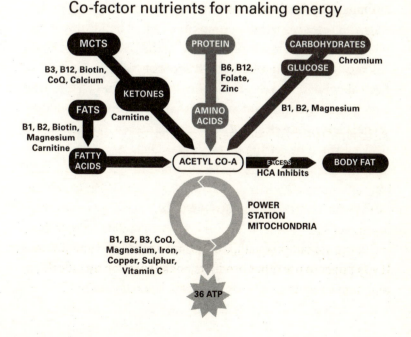

There are three nutrients that are worth a special mention: carnitine, hydroxycitric acid (HCA), found in garcinia cambogia, which is a type of tamarind, and chromium – the nutrients contained in GL Support.

The minerals zinc and magnesium are important too. Zinc, as well as triggering autophagy, is very important for digestion, helping to make digestive enzymes as well as stomach acid[1], and for detoxification. Zinc is rich in seeds and nuts, but is worth supplementing. Aim for 15mg a day, the amount often provided in good multivitamins.

Magnesium is key to your metabolism as it's needed by the majority of the enzymes in your body. It also helps muscles to relax and it's a key nutrient to support detoxification. It is also a vital part of the energy-making cycle inside mitochondria and is vital for both fat and carbohydrate metabolism, as well as being essential for nerve cells to send their messages – in other words, your brain function. It has also been shown to trigger autophagy in animal studies.[2] Magnesium is rich in greens, nuts and seeds, especially pumpkin. A small handful will give you about 75mg. The average intake in the UK is 272mg. If you eat your greens and seeds, you'll probably take in 350mg. We need about 450mg a day for optimal health, so it's wise to take a daily multivitamin and mineral that gives you at least 100mg of magnesium as well as eating magnesium-rich foods. That will be what you'll be getting on the 5-Day Diet.

Epsom salts

There's a good way of getting the benefits of magnesium: an Epsom salt bath. Epsom salts are magnesium sulphate. Both sulphur and magnesium

▶

help detoxification, and Epsom salts alkalise and help to reduce pain. A lot of the toxins that the body eliminates during a fast are acid. During my retreats I recommend an Epsom salt bath using 500–600g of Epsom salts (a cupful) and staying in the bath for 10 minutes. This has been shown to raise blood levels of magnesium.[3] (See Resources for a supplier of pure Epsom salts without perfumes or other chemicals.)

Carnitine – essential for ketosis

Carnitine is a semi-essential nutrient. This means that although your body can make it, it doesn't necessarily make enough for optimal health, especially when you're burning fat, which increases the need for it. Carnitine is vital both for burning fats and for feeding fats into the ketogenic fire. You can help to guarantee the conversion of fats into energy by supplementing with extra carnitine.

Carnitine combines with fats to deliver them into the cell's mitochondria for burning. It's called the 'carnitine shuttle' because, once the fat is delivered, carnitine is shuttled back to do it again.

Ideally, it's better to take carnitine three times a day because it only hangs around in your body for a few hours. During the 5-Day Diet I recommend that you take carnitine, which is included in GL Support, three times a day, with each meal, which is when you need it most.

Hydroxycitric acid – the Thai secret?

Thailand, and South-East Asia in general, has one of the lowest rates of obesity, diabetes, cancer and heart disease. The Thai diet has many redeeming factors, and one is the widespread use of tamarind fruit, the rind of which, known as garcinia cambogia, contains hydroxycitric acid, or HCA, which makes it harder for the body to turn sugar into fat. When you consume more carbs than you need, your body's metabolism can shunt the excess to make more fats, which then get stored, and more cholesterol. The critical enzyme in this fat-producing pathway is called ATP-citrate lyase and is partially inhibited by the HCA in garcinia cambogia. Dampening down this enzyme reduces LDL cholesterol, a fatty liver and inflammation, heart-disease risk and blood sugar problems associated with diabetes in animal studies.[4] It also cranks up the thyroid, thus telling the body to make more energy, instead of storing it as fat.[5] In one study fat rats given HCA lost significant amounts of weight, and improved blood sugar control and reduced inflammation.[6] It also reduces appetite, possibly by giving serotonin levels a boost. It also triggers autophagy, as we learnt in Part 1.

Hydroxycitric acid is clearly effective for weight loss when given in the right dose, the most effective dose in studies being 2,300mg a day: for example, 750mg taken three times a day. A meta-analysis of nine good-quality trials confirms a significant weight loss in the order of 1.2kg (2.7lb) in eight weeks.[7] Best results have been reported in trials giving over 2g a day, averaging 3.5kg (8lb) weight loss over 8 weeks or 0.5kg (1lb) a week. As an example, a trial put 60 volunteers on a 2,000-calorie diet, plus a 30-minute walking exercise programme five days a week and gave them either a placebo or 2,800mg of HCA in three equally divided doses 30–60 minutes before meals. At the end of eight weeks, body weight had dropped by 5.4 per cent in those taking HCA compared to placebo and their body mass index (BMI) decreased by 5.2 per cent. Food intake, total cholesterol, LDL (the bad guy), triglycerides and serum leptin levels (the hormone that triggers eating) were significantly reduced, while HDL cholesterol (the good guy), serotonin levels and excretion of urinary fat metabolites (a biomarker of fat oxidation) significantly increased. No significant adverse effects were reported.[8]

Any downsides? There have been some case reports of potential liver toxicity; however, they have been in people with diabetes or fatty liver disease or on potentially liver-toxic medication or extremely low-calorie diets, so it's hard to know if HCA had anything to do with this. No downsides have been reported in healthy people supplementing only HCA. A major review deemed it safe, certainly up to 2,800mg a day,[9] which is enough to support weight loss. Animal studies and clinical investigations have not found evidence of potential harm: 'In both animal and clinical literature, elevated intakes of HCA per se have not led to signs of inflammation or hepatotoxicity. The compound has been found to reduce markers of inflammation in brain, intestines, kidney and serum,' reports Dr Harry Preuss, director of the American College of Nutrition. Even so, I would err on the side of caution, if you have any liver dysfunction or non-alcoholic fatty liver disease, in taking it in the long-term.

In order to benefit from the diet, I recommend that you take 2,250mg of HCA, in three divided doses with meals, during the 5-Day Diet.

Chromium - the sugar stabiliser

The older you are, the less likely you are to be taking in enough chromium[10] – an essential mineral that helps to stabilise blood sugar levels by making you more sensitive to insulin.[11] It contributes to normal nutrient metabolism and to the maintenance of normal blood glucose levels. Presumably, as a consequence, supplementing chromium has been shown to reduce appetite and promote weight loss,[12] reduce PMS-related mood dips[13] and depression,[14] and reduce fatigue in diabetics.[15] The average daily intake is below 50mcg, whereas an optimal intake, certainly for those with blood sugar concerns, is around 200mcg. The results of a recent meta-analysis of 22 trials reported a normalisation of blood glucose, HbA1c, cholesterol (LDL down, HDL up) and triglycerides with more than 200mcg a day.[16] You'll be receiving 235mcg a day during the 5-Day Diet.

Chromium is found in wholefoods, whole grains, beans, nuts and seeds. Asparagus and mushrooms are especially rich in chromium, both of which are included in this diet. Chromium works with insulin to help stabilise your blood sugar level, so when you feel stressed and have erratic energy, you use up more, and therefore you have a greater need for chromium. Hence someone with a sugar and stimulant addiction, eating a diet high in refined foods, is most at risk of deficiency. White flour has 98 per cent of its chromium removed in the refining process – another reason to stay away from refined foods.

Chapter 9

Monitoring Your Ketones, Glucose and Progress

You will have your own reasons for wanting to follow the 5-Day Diet. For some it is for weight loss and for others there will be health reasons – wanting more energy being the most common. For most people it is both.

Monitoring changes: weight, measurements, ketosis

If you have access to a set of bathroom scales and a tape measure, it's easy to measure your weight before and after, your waist and hip measurements, and the ratio between the two. Your waist:hip ratio is a good indicator of a healthy weight. The ideal ratio in healthy pre-menopausal women ranges between 0.67

and 0.8. This ratio reflects waists between 61cm and 71cm (24in and 28in) with 92cm (36in) hips, and waists between 69cm and 79cm (27in and 31in) with 102cm (40in) hips. For men the ideal waist:hip ratio is between 0.85 and 0.95.

If you have access to a body-fat composition monitor you can also monitor your before-and-after body fat percentage. Please note, though, that these are very approximate and you might not pick up much apparent change in five days, so don't be disheartened. If you are losing weight, you will be burning fat. There are 'Monitor your progress' charts at the back of the book to add these measurements.

When you go into ketosis, you'll burn off your sugar stores, which are held as glycogen (sugar plus water) and hence you lose water, as explained in the Introduction. This will look like weight loss on the scales, but what you want is *fat* loss. I recommend that you don't weigh yourself until the end of Day 6, or even Day 7, when you're back to eating carbs, although in moderation. Your body will quickly replenish glycogen stores, so the difference between your before and after weights will more accurately reflect fat loss, which is what you want. It takes less than 24 hours to reload glycogen stores when you begin eating carbs again.

Glucose and ketone levels

During my retreats my team also monitors glucose and ketone levels. This is easy to do but it does require buying a monitor to use at home. I've made a film showing how all these monitors work, vieweable in the 'resources and testing' section on www. hybriddiet.co.uk. A number of meters are now available that allow you to measure your blood glucose and ketones in the comfort of your own home. Those meters that use individual ketone and glucose strips range in price from £10 to £25, with the more expensive versions usually including some of the strips, which otherwise have to be bought separately. However, the cost soon adds up when you run out of strips and have to buy more, because each replacement ketone strip can cost anywhere from £1 to £3, depending on the brand. You also have the inconvenience of probably having to prick your finger twice for each strip, or juggling two strips, resetting the meter in between.

The KEYA Smart Meter

A simpler alternative – and one that is certainly more cost-effective over the long term – is the KEYA Smart Meter (see Resources), which measures both glucose and ketones after a drop of blood is added to a single strip. This is what we use on our Hybrid Fast Detox Retreats. The best deal is a package that includes 110 strips – enough for more than three months of daily tests, meaning that you can test your daily glucose and ketone scores for as little as a £1.35 a day. By the end of that period, you'll be the master of your metabolism. In the figure below you can see the average increase in blood ketones and the drop in blood glucose that we see on our retreats.

Glucose, ketones and the GKI (glucose ketone index)

	Day 1	Day 2	Day 3	Day 4	Day 5	Day 6
Ketones (mmol/l)	1.6	2.4	3.1	2.95	4.7	1.2
Glucose (mmol/l)	6.1	5.8	5.2	4.8	4.4	7.1
GKI	3.8	2.4	1.7	1.6	0.9	5.9

As soon as your ketone level is above 0.5mmol/l you're heading into ketosis. Ideally, you want to get to a score of between 2 and 5mmol/l. Also, you'll see your glucose level start to drop, to ideally below 5, ending up below 5mmol/l and above 3mmol/l by the fifth day. If you are diabetic, you'll probably be at the higher end of this range.

Don't measure your glucose level after exercise, as your body will make glucose to enable exercise, be it from glycogen stores, fat or protein. Also, don't measure immediately after a meal. The best time to measure is before a meal; for example, before lunch if you exercised before your Hybrid Latté, or before dinner if you exercised before lunch. Afterwards, measure your ketone and glucose scores at the same time every day.

You can work out your own GKI (glucose ketone index) by dividing your glucose score by your ketone score. You are aiming for your GKI to be reducing every day. Once you're below 2 (where glucose is no more than double the ketones) you're in the zone. But bear in mind that this relates to blood ketone levels. If you measure ketones in breath (using a ketone breath monitor, see below) the figures won't exactly correlate, so the important thing is to see your GKI reduce every day.

There are 'Monitor your progress' charts at the back of this book for recording your glucose and ketone scores during the 5-Day Diet (see page 190).

Ketone breath monitors

Alternatively, you can measure ketones in breath using a breathalyser. This is a different kind of ketone (acetone) to that found in the blood (beta-hydroxybutyrate or BHB) so the figures won't compare exactly. If you are using a breathalyser (there are two available called Ketonix Breath Test and Ketoscan Mini) the important thing is simply to check that you are registering with breath ketones. Both monitors have a range to indicate that you're in ketosis.

These monitors are the easiest and cheapest way to measure ketones, because you don't need to keep pricking your finger and buying test strips.

Ketonix consists of the measuring device and a rechargeable battery pack. Alternatively, it can be powered through a computer's USB port. The reading is transmitted to, and stored by, an app on a smartphone or computer. The main part of the display is a dial (like a speedometer), with blue, green, yellow and red regions. Blue (0–4 parts per million or ppm) means that you are not in ketosis; green (4–30ppm) means you are; and red (above 80ppm) means that your level of ketones is dangerously high.

The system is easy to use (although it takes about ten minutes to reboot if you have unplugged the battery pack). A greater concern is its accuracy, because you can get different readings depending on how you breathe into the tube. Acetone tends to accumulate in the lowest part of the lungs, so the instructions are to blow out every last millilitre of air, then to keep exhaling until you are almost gasping. This is hard to do at first, but you'll get used to it – make sure you use the same technique every time.

Acetone in the breath is a fair reflection of beta-hydroxybutyrate in the blood but the measurement is different, so don't expect the same actual numbers as a ketone blood test.

Ketoscan Mini is easier to use and has the advantage of giving you a reading on the device itself. It also seems to be more consistent, and less dependent on exactly how you exhale. The instructions say 'take a deep breath in then exhale into the device'. It also measures in parts per million (ppm) and says that above 5ppm you're clearly in ketosis. This is comparable to Ketonix. It also links to an app for tracking your progress.

The one disadvantage of the Ketoscan Mini is that you have to buy a new cartridge after 300 tests. Overall, it works out at less than 13p a test, with an initial outlay of around £150, much like the Ketonix.

See Resources for suppliers and the best offers.

How to monitor your health issues

How is your energy level? If ten out of ten was the best energy level you have ever experienced or can imagine, and zero out of ten the worst, where are you now? On the day before you start your 5-Day Diet, pick a number as an average of how your energy has been for the week before that day, then write this in the 'Monitor your progress' chart on page 190. Then, do the same thing on the day after the diet, Day 6. Also, do this one week later, marked as 'week after' – many people experience a big increase in energy in the following weeks.

Now, pick two other health concerns. It could be your digestion, your sleep, your level of stress or anxiety, your mood or your pain, with ten out of ten being no pain and zero out of ten being the worst. Again, score these at the start and end of the five days using the chart on page 190.

I'd love to know how you fare, and it is very helpful for ongoing research, so, if you can, please take a photograph (or a scan) of your results and send them to me at patrick@patrickholford. com, putting 'hybrid results' in the title.

Your ideal glycosylated haemoglobin level

If you are diabetic, pre-diabetic or concerned about your blood sugar, the level of glycosylated haemoglobin in the blood is the best long-term indicator of problems with blood sugar control. It measures HbA1c which, put simply, is the number of red blood cells that have become sugar damaged. Because red blood cells live for about three months, it's a long-term measure of your blood sugar resilience, in other words how good your body is at bringing high blood sugar spikes down. A high percentage of glycosylated red blood cells, therefore, indicates a high number of sugar spikes over the previous three-month period. If your glycosylated haemoglobin is more than 7 per cent (53mmol/mol), the chances are that you already have diabetes or will soon develop it. The HbA1c should be below 5.6 per cent (or 37mmol/mol) in a healthy body. The table below shows how to interpret your results.

How to interpret your HbA1c results

Healthy	Not great	Dysglycemia	Diabetes
<5.6 per cent	5.6–6.5 per cent	>6.5 per cent	>7 per cent
<37mmol/mol	37–48mmol/mol	>49mmol/mol	>53mmol/mol

Your doctor will conduct this test if he or she is concerned that you might have diabetes, or it might be included in a more advanced blood 'work up'. You can also buy a home test kit and do it yourself (see Resources).

Unlike glucose, your level of HbA1c does not change

overnight, which makes it a much more accurate indicator of diabetes; however, this also means that it takes a while to see any significant improvement after altering your diet. And it will be three months before you see the full effect.

I therefore recommend doing this before starting the 5-Day Diet and then three months later when you've either completed one to three cycles or adopted a low-GL diet with much less carbs.

Although HbA1c is a very valuable and informative test, it will not tell you if or when you have entered ketosis in the high-fat phase. For that, you will need to conduct a blood or breath analysis of your ketone levels, as described above.

Chapter 10

Troubleshooting Q&A

Q: I'm really craving something sweet – what do you advise?

Don't skip any of the meals and snacks. Do drink your 500ml Carboslow/Immune C drink, into which you can add a tea-spoon of Blueberry Active. Keeping yourself hydrated will reduce your appetite. If you're still desperate, have a teaspoon of Ketofast (C8 oil). Your body treats this as fuel and turns off your appetite. Your desire for sweet foods will reduce dramatically during the 5-Day Diet.

Q: What if I experience a headache?

When your blood sugar level dips and you start to switch over to running on ketones in the first 48 hours, it can trigger a headache. Headaches can also occur if you are withdrawing from caffeine and also if you are detoxifying. Make sure you are drinking enough water, have an Epsom salt bath (see page 96) but also consider taking 100mg of niacin (vitamin B3) in the blushing form, together with a painkiller. Do not buy the 'no blush' form of niacin. The blush, which lasts for about 20 minutes, is a vasodilation and helps both to detoxify the body and can relieve headaches. You will feel warm when the flushing starts and a bit cold when it ends. Either have a hot bath as you start to feel colder, or lie down and keep warm. The after-effects of niacin can be very calming and muscle relaxing, and you might fall asleep. This is good. The chances are you'll wake up without a headache.

Q: I'm constipated

This can happen if you have a particularly sluggish system, and you eat little without enough fibre and water. This is why it is vital to have 1.5 litres of the Carboslow and ImmuneC drink. If you are already doing this, you can assist elimination by taking up to three capsules a day of Blessed Herbs Digestive Stimulator capsules (see Resources). Also do the udiyanna bandha exercise on page 48, and take a brisk walk each day.

Q: My ketones have gone very high

If you are reading in the red zone on either of the ketone breathalysers, this is not good; however, there are reasons why this might be a false reading. If you have had any alcohol, this will create a false high. Also, it's best to do the breath test away from food or any drink – ideally 15 minutes or more after consuming anything.

If you have type-1 diabetes, and both your glucose levels and ketones are high, this is a sign that you do not have sufficient insulin. This can cause an abnormal production of ketones, called ketoacidosis. This is unlikely to happen from fasting, or on this diet, unless you are a type-1 diabetic. If this does happen, contact your doctor.

Q: My glucose has gone very low

Many glucose monitors will start to say you have 'low' glucose below 4 mmol/l but this can and does occur in some people on the 5-Day Diet. If your glucose is below 4 and your ketone level is high, for example above 3, this simply means that you are burning ketones instead of glucose. This is not dangerous.

Q: Can I take my medication while doing this diet?

I do not recommend that anyone with type-2 diabetes combines this diet with any other medication than metformin. If you are on other medication, please ask your doctor if it is safe for you to do this diet and make sure you have a point of contact to discuss your test results as the diet progresses. The same applies with type-1 diabetes. You need medical back-up to support you during this diet. Other medication should not be a problem, but it is worth checking first with your medical practitioner.

Q: What if I'm not losing weight?

The two most common causes for not losing weight are an underlying thyroid problem or an unidentified food intolerance. The thyroid gland produces thyroxine, the hormone that speeds up your metabolism. If you find it really hard to lose weight and also feel cold, or you have poor temperature tolerance and sluggish digestion, it is well worth getting your thyroid hormone levels checked. A low level of thyroxine and a high level of thyroid-stimulating hormone (TSH) indicates that you have an underactive thyroid. Once treated there is no reason not to succeed on this diet.

Weight gain is a common reaction to foods we're intolerant to. Most of us have intolerances or allergies to certain foods, but few of us are aware of them. It follows, then, that eliminating the food that you are unknowingly intolerant to can lead to highly dramatic weight loss. But not all allergies or food intolerances are for life. The most extreme allergies involve the body producing an IgE antibody against the food. These sensitivities stay for life. But most food intolerances involve the IgG type of antibody. If you avoid the identified food(s) strictly for three to four months, your IgG antibodies will die off and they don't pass on that memory to the next generation, so you can grow out of this kind of intolerance. This means that you can reintroduce previously problematic foods back into your diet. If you think you are food sensitive or allergic, it is best to have a proper quantitative IgG ELISA test (see Resources).

Water retention, bloating and puffiness are all common types of reactions, and they make you feel and look fatter. Once you've singled out and eliminated the foods that are triggering your intolerant response, you are likely to see dramatic changes very quickly. It's not unusual to lose up to 3kg (7lb) within three or four days.

Apart from weight gain and bloating, food allergies and intolerances also cause other problems, such as aches and pains, headaches, fatigue, mood swings, and annoying skin and digestive conditions. These also go when you identify and avoid what you are allergic or intolerant to.

If you have any other questions during the diet, you can post them on my Facebook page. If you are a 100% Health Club member we have a private Facebook group for questions and sharing results.

Part 3

Transitioning to a Low-GL Diet

As explained earlier in the book, the best diet for you to follow after completing the 5-Day Diet is my low-GL diet for either continued weight loss or as a lifestyle. I also advise you to follow it for a couple of days before starting the five days to give your body the best chance for quick results. The lifestyle diet is not a diet as such, but a way of life. It is your basic diet for keeping yourself healthy, full of life and free of disease. This part explains how.

Chapter 11

Eating Low-GL for Life – The Principles

Whenever I'm asked what the ideal diet for life should be, I answer that it is a low-GL (low-glycaemic load) diet. By definition this is a diet that keeps your blood sugar level even, as I explained in the box on page 54. This means that you produce little insulin, which is not only the fat-storing hormone but also a promoter, in excess, of cancer cell growth and numerous other diseases, from heart disease to diabetes, and from dementia to depression.

There are more immediate benefits as well, however, such as increased energy throughout the day, and better and more consistent concentration and mood. Below are examples of the feedback I receive on a regular basis from people embarking on my low-GL diet:

'I feel incredible. Before, I didn't have a cut-off switch. Now I feel full and can leave food on the plate because I'm full.' Adrian

'It's as if someone has given me a magic pill and said, "You'll have more energy, you'll feel calm and you'll feel less stressed." I am full of energy.' Marianne

'This is the easiest way to lose weight and stay healthy I've ever tried.' Glynda

'My energy level is incredible. My blood sugar is well under control (I'm diabetic). It's been so easy.' Linda

'I lost 6kg (13lb) in a month and, amazingly, I lost my craving for sweets! My energy level increased so much.' John

You might have already experienced some of these benefits, both on the 5-Day Diet and in the days following it, because it is then that your renewed energy factories, the mitochondria, start making energy. Rest assured that these kinds of benefits will continue, and, over the longer term, you'll also be reducing your risk of suffering with the majority of the 21st-century diseases, or reversing these diseases if you already have one of them.

The glycaemic load of foods, and why they are important to know

As we saw on page 54, the GL of a food or a meal is a precise measurement made by knowing two things: how many carbs you are eating (for example, one or three slices of toast) and how fast-releasing the sugar is in that food (slow-releasing wholegrain rye sourdough bread v. fast-releasing white bread, for example). The speed of release of sugars, called the GI (glycaemic index) is influenced by how much fibre there is in the food and what kind of sugar is in the food. Berries, for example, have a lot of xylose, which is a slow-releasing sugar, whereas grapes and raisins have a lot of glucose, which is fast-releasing. By multiplying the quantity or amount of carbs by the quality, or GI score, you get the GL score. (You don't have to do this maths, though, because I've done it for you.) My preferred low-GL diet, as you'll see in this part, provides 60 GLs to maintain weight and 45 GLs if you want to continue losing weight after the 5-Day Diet. This is described as a low-GL diet. On the 5-Day Diet, in contrast, you've been eating under 15 GLs, as it's a very low-carb diet (and very low calorie, too).

Which diet is best?

There's a bit of a debate about whether my kind of low-GL diet – that still includes carbs, although slow-releasing and in controlled amounts – or a very low-carb, high-fat ketogenic diet works best for weight control and diabetes. This debate is the subject of *The Hybrid Diet* book in which I and my co-author Jerome Burne effectively conclude that:

- There are some conditions, such as neurodegenerative diseases, where a very low-carb, ketogenic diet works best.

- It's probably best for all of us to switch from time to time, which is what doing the 5-Day Diet achieves, but eat my kind of a low-GL diet as your baseline lifestyle diet.

- Different people prefer, and probably function better, on different diets, so at least you have a choice. Meat lovers, for example, often prefer the high-fat, low-carb type of diet whereas vegetarians and vegans do better on my kind of low-GL diet, although the diet is also suitable for those who prefer to eat smaller quantities of meat or poultry.

- Both approaches work better than the conventional low-fat, high-carb calorie-controlled diet for weight loss.

A low-GL diet prevents and reverses disease

More than any other criterion, the GL of your diet associates with a lower risk of just about every disease you're likely to suffer from. Also, lowering the GL of your diet has been shown to *reverse* many diseases as well. It is also the best predictor of how much insulin you are going to produce in response to a meal (it works better than knowing the grams of carbs), which we have learnt is critical, not only for health, but also for triggering autophagy and reducing cancer cell growth.

These are the benefits:

- Prevention and reversal of weight gain.

- Less hunger and sugar cravings.

- Better appetite control and weight-loss maintenance.

- Prevention and reversal of diabetes,

- Prevention and reversal of heart disease, hypertension (high blood pressure) and high cholesterol.

- Reduction in the risk of cancers of the breast, prostate,

colon and rectum, ovary, thyroid, endometrium
and pancreas.

- Reduction in Alzheimer's dementia risk and cognitive
impairment.

- Reduction in depression and aggression, and improvement
in stress resilience.

- Switches on anti-ageing genes.

- It lowers IGF-1, associated with accelerating ageing and
increasing cancer risk.

The evidence from studies for all these is discussed in detail in
The Hybrid Diet for those who wish to delve into the science.
There's another layer of evidence in relation to specific common
diseases in my books *Say No to Heart Disease*, *Say No to Cancer*,
Say No to Diabetes, *The Alzheimer's Prevention Plan*, *The Feel
Good Factor* (about depression) and *The Stress Cure*. If these are
your particular concerns, you might want to dig deeper, as these
books cover other critical factors that drive these diseases, and
how to reverse them.

For now, let's get stuck into how you actually eat a low-GL
diet, starting with the fundamental principles.

The principles of the low-GL diet

There are four core principles at the heart of my low-GL diet.
Each of them is a positive guideline in its own right, and each
supports the others. They are easy to attain and essential if you
are serious about achieving permanent weight loss and 100 per
cent health.

1. Balance your blood sugar by eating 45 GLs a day for weight loss or 60 GLs for maintaining health.

2. Eat good fats, and avoid bad fats.

3. Supplement for success (see Chapter 13).

4. Keep on the move – exercise is important (see Chapter 14).

Why should you balance your blood sugar?

Balancing your blood sugar, and consequently keeping your insulin level down, is the fundamental concept at the heart of the low-GL diet. Once your blood sugar and insulin levels are in balance, sustainable weight loss (if you're on 45 GLs a day) and better health will follow, and will continue when following the higher-GL lifestyle diet of 60 GLs. Success is inevitable.

Keeping your blood sugar balanced depends not only on what you eat, but also on how and when you eat. Later in this chapter I'll explain exactly which foods and food combinations stabilise your blood sugar best and help to burn fat. When you understand that it is high-GL foods and meals that lead to gaining weight, you'll understand how to control what you eat to lose weight, or to maintain your healthy weight.

In time GL-awareness will become second nature, and before you know it you'll be experimenting by mixing and matching your own combinations of low-GL foods at every meal. Reducing your blood sugar level will encourage fat burning instead of fat storing; your appetite will be satisfied and you will feel energetic for longer than you are used to. Knowing your GL will become a lifestyle essential.

The first step in the low-GL direction is to avoid adding sugar, or foods with added sugar, as well as avoiding refined carbohydrates, which tend to be white in colour: white bread, rice and pasta, for example. The unrefined carbohydrates are better for you because they are turned into glucose slowly, and your body has more time to use the energy. They tend to be brown in colour, providing more fibre: brown rice, whole grains, brown bread and wholewheat pasta, for example. Eating too many unrefined carbohydrates increases your blood sugar levels fast – which produces excess glucose, which turns into fat.

The carbs at a glance

The key factor to remember is to control the glycaemic load (GL) of the carbs you eat – 10 GLs for weight loss or 15 GLs for maintenance for a main meal and 5 GLs for a snack. This won't make sense just yet, but it will do by the time you've read this chapter.

Neither fat nor protein substantially affects blood sugar, but carbs do, so you need to prioritise eating slow (low-GL) carbs in the right quantity to optimise your health, weight and energy.

In visual terms, half your plate will comprise vegetables and/or low-GL fruit, one-quarter of the plate will be protein-rich foods and one-quarter carbohydrate-rich foods as shown overleaf. If you prefer to think in terms of calories, this equates to about 20 per cent of your total calorific intake from protein, 30 per cent from fat and 50 per cent from carbohydrates – but you won't be counting calories. The focus is not on fats so there is no need to avoid the healthy fats in nuts and seeds, their oils and oily fish, and it wouldn't matter if you increased your fat intake, as long as you reduce your carb intake accordingly.

The low-GL food plate

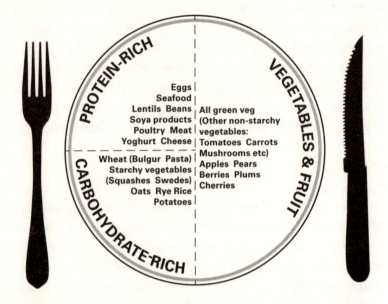

Aim for 45 GLs a day for weight loss, distributed evenly throughout the day: 10 GLs in each of the three main meals, two 5-GL snacks (mid-morning and late afternoon), plus an additional 5 GLs for drinks and/or desserts. For lifestyle, or maintenance, aim for 60 GLs a day, distributed evenly throughout the day: 15 GLs in each of the three main meals) two 5-GL snacks (mid-morning and late afternoon), plus an additional 5GLs for drinks and/or desserts.

This way you will be able to have a low-GL dessert, diluted fruit juice or even a small glass of dry white wine or spirit.

What to eat for breakfast

When you wake up, your blood sugar is low because you haven't eaten for hours, so you need to give your body some fuel unless you're purposely fasting. This could be a low-GL breakfast such as eggs with oatcakes or Scandinavian-style rye bread (pumpernickel), or perhaps porridge oats with chia seeds and berries. (If you want to, you can also add a bit of intermittent fasting by having a Hybrid Latté as your breakfast, thus having an 18-hour food fast if you ate dinner at 6pm or 7pm and then have lunch at noon or 1pm the next day, as I explained in Chapter 5.)

Some people think that they will eat less and lose weight if they avoid eating throughout the morning; however, this idea has been put to the test and not found to be true. One group of volunteers ate three meals and two snacks at the traditional times, while another ate exactly the same food between noon and 11pm. The delayed eaters gained more weight and had a less healthy metabolism.[1] Another study found that establishing a routine in which you eat at regular intervals throughout the daylight hours allows your metabolism to adjust and provide all the energy you need.[2]

If you struggle with fluctuating energy levels, therefore, and you tend to fall asleep during the day, or if you find it difficult to lose weight, switch to the daily regime of three meals and two snacks. This will help you to avoid an all-too-familiar scenario: you try to prop yourself up with liquid stimulants (coffee or tea), nicotine or instant sugar in the form of a piece of toast or a croissant, but the resolve to go without food still weakens as your blood sugar dips lower and lower. Finally, you buckle under the strain and end up bingeing on high-GL foods.

This is why you must eat a healthy breakfast. But what should you eat and how much? Nutritionists gave one group of children a low-GL breakfast and another group a high-GL breakfast, then allowed both groups free access to a buffet lunch. Although both groups declared that they were satisfied immediately after breakfast, at lunchtime the high-GL group were hungrier and ate more food.[3] Another study reported exactly the same result in adults.[4]

The message is clear: eat a low-GL breakfast. It will satisfy you for longer by keeping your blood sugar more stable, so you will eat less later. There are two ways to do this:

1. Simply choose any of the low-GL breakfasts starting on page 154. Each of these gives you sufficient protein and essential fats but no more than 10 GL of carbs.

2. Alternatively, 'do it yourself', using the chart below as a guide.

Low-GL breakfast guidelines

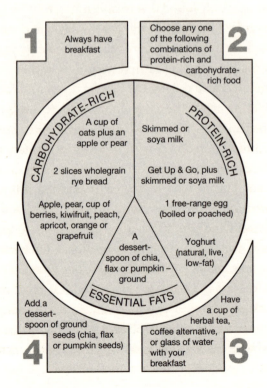

1 Always have breakfast

2 Choose any one of the following combinations of protein-rich and carbohydrate-rich food

CARBOHYDRATE-RICH

A cup of oats plus an apple or pear

2 slices wholegrain rye bread

Apple, pear, cup of berries, kiwifruit, peach, apricot, orange or grapefruit

PROTEIN-RICH

Skimmed or soya milk

Get Up & Go, plus skimmed or soya milk

1 free-range egg (boiled or poached)

Yoghurt (natural, live, low-fat)

A dessertspoon of chia, flax or pumpkin – ground

ESSENTIAL FATS

4 Add a dessertspoon of ground seeds (chia, flax or pumpkin seeds)

3 Have a cup of herbal tea, coffee alternative, or glass of water with your breakfast

The following breakfasts will give you the perfect balance of carbohydrate and protein:

Low-GL breakfasts

Carbohydrates	+	Protein
Cereal/fruit	+	Seeds/yoghurt/milk
Fruit	+	Yoghurt/seeds
Fruit	+	Get Up & Go with CarboSlow/milk
Bread/toast	+	Egg
Bread/toast	+	Fish (such as kippers)

Get Up & Go breakfasts

One of the simplest and best breakfasts is the original Get Up & Go. It's a delicious powder made from a variety of whole foods, including quinoa, oats, seeds, almonds and cinnamon, with lots of added vitamins and minerals, such as vitamin C (1,000mg per portion), B vitamins and chromium (50mcg per portion), all of which are essential for a healthy metabolism.

It's guaranteed to fill you up until lunchtime, yet each serving is only 283 calories and 5 GLs, so you could blend it with 5 GLs of strawberries, raspberries, pear or blackcurrants for a healthy, balanced breakfast. A teaspoon of cinnamon will make this shake extra tasty. Alternatively, add a scoop of Get Up & Go to two cups of milk or carb-free almond milk and a handful of berries. (Frozen berries defrost almost instantly in a blender.)

An even better and even lower GL version is Get Up & Go with CarboSlow, which you met on the 5-Day Diet. It includes 1g of super-soluble glucomannan fibre (see page 44) in each serving. Or you can buy CarboSlow separately and add it to original Get Up & Go yourself (see Resources). A serving of Get Up & Go with CarboSlow, plus berries and carb-free almond milk, is just 6 GLs (or 8 GLs if you use oat milk), which is why I include a smaller portion in the 5-Day Diet. Equally, because it is perfectly balanced for protein, carbs, vitamins and minerals, you could simply drink a glass three times a day during the weight-loss diet phase after the 5-Day Diet if you want to keep losing weight, which would see you cruising along on a mere 21 GLs (well below your 45-GL allowance); however, this would leave you deficient in omega-3 fats, so I recommend adding a dessertspoon of chia seeds and/or taking a fish oil supplement.

Cereal breakfasts

If you prefer a more traditional cereal-, fruit- or toast-based breakfast, there are a few points to consider.

First, any cereal-based breakfast must include a low-GL cereal and low-GL fruit as a sweetener, plus sufficient protein and essential fats. Remember, the goal is to consume no more than 10 GLs. If you don't need to lose weight, you can increase the carb portion to 15 GLs. In practical terms, just make sure your portions of the breakfasts below fill you up.

Each of the portions in the table below provides 5 GLs. As you can see, the best 'value', in terms of satisfying your hunger, are oat flakes, either cooked (as in porridge) or eaten raw (like cornflakes). Basically, you can eat as much as you like, given that two servings will fill up anybody.

Cereal breakfasts

Cereal	Serving size
Oat flakes	2 servings or cups
All-Bran	1 serving (½ bowl or 1 cup)
Unsweetened muesli	1 small serving (less than ½ bowl or ¾ cup)
Alpen	½ serving (¼ bowl or ½ cup)
Raisin Bran	½ serving (¼ bowl or ½ cup)
Weetabix	1 biscuit

Tip: Adding a spoonful of oat bran will lower the GL of any cereal.

Obviously, these cereals can be quite dull on their own, so you might want to consider adding fruit. Again, each of the portions in the table below is equivalent to 5 GLs.

Low-GL fruits

Fruit	Serving size
Berries	1 large punnet
Pear	1
Grapefruit	1
Apple	1 small (fits into the palm of your hand)
Peach	1 small
Banana	Less than half

To keep hunger at bay, your best option would be porridge (or raw oat flakes) with as many berries as you could eat. Alternatively, you could have half a bowl of All-Bran and a grapefruit, or half a bowl of unsweetened muesli with a small apple.

As far as protein is concerned, there is some in both milk and soya milk (but always pick the unsweetened kind). Rice milk is high GL so it is best avoided. Oat milk is not bad, but not as good as soya. Yoghurt (unsweetened and well fermented, which gives it a bitter taste) is roughly the same as milk or soya milk, so feel free to have a spoonful on your cereal.

Seeds are another good source of protein, and they also contain countless vitamins, minerals, essential fats and fibre. I recommend a tablespoon of ground seeds or chopped nuts on your cereal. Chia seeds are the best choice, because they are high in both protein and soluble fibre. Also, you don't have to grind them because they have a soft outer husk. If you leave your cereal and chia for a few minutes, the seeds will soften and be less crunchy when you eat them. Flax seeds are the next best option, but they are not as tasty. Pumpkin seeds are good, too, and high in magnesium.

The best cereal-based breakfast is Low-GL Granola (see page 156), which is made by mixing half oat flakes with Lizi's Low-GL Granola (purchased), seeds and fresh berries. One serving (8 GLs) is completely satisfying.

Yoghurt breakfasts

If you are especially fond of yoghurt, you could dispense with the cereal and just have yoghurt, fruit and seeds. Each of the following portions provides about 5 GLs, assuming that a small pot is 150g:

Yoghurts

Yoghurt	Serving size
Plain yoghurt	2 small pots, 300g
Non-fat yoghurt	2 small pots, 300g
Low-fat yoghurt with added fruit and sugar	⅔ small pot, 100g

Providing you choose a yoghurt that has no added sugar, you can eat two small pots, sweeten it with any of the fruits from the previous table and add a tablespoon of ground seeds. There is absolutely no need to go for the low-fat option. Unsweetened coconut yogurt is a good choice for those avoiding dairy.

Egg and toast breakfasts

Half the calories in every egg come from fat, but the type of fat depends on what the chicken has been fed; for example, eggs from intensively reared chickens are high in saturated fat. Fortunately, though, most free-range chickens are fed much healthier diets that provide a healthier balance of fats.

Unsurprisingly, omega-3-rich free-range or organic eggs are much better for you than ordinary eggs, but I still recommend that you eat no more than six of these a week; for example, you could have either two small or one large egg for breakfast every other day. Poach, boil or scramble them, because the high heat of frying damages the essential fats.

As eggs are pure protein and fat (and therefore 0 GL), you could combine them with any of the following:

Breads and oatcakes

Food	Serving size	
	10 GL	**15 GL**
Oatcakes	4	6
Pumpernickel (unyeasted rye bread)	2 thin slices	3 thin slices
Sourdough rye bread	2 thin slices	2 slices
Wholemeal rye bread (yeasted)	1 slice	1.5 slices
Wholemeal wheat bread (yeasted)	1 slice	1.5 slices

Even high-fibre white bread is best avoided, as just one slice would see you exceeding 10 GLs. I recommend oatcakes, Scandinavian-style pumpernickel, sonnenbrot- or volkornbrot-type breads, or yeast-free sourdough rye bread instead. All sourdough breads are substantial, flavoursome and high in fibre. By contrast, light, white, fluffy 'fake' breads are full of air, super-refined and nutritionally inferior. My simple rule of thumb is the squish factor: the squishier the bread the higher the GL.

Making the switch to 'real' bread might be a bit of a shock at first, but you'll soon discover that it is much more satisfying as well as healthier. Real breads are sometimes made from grains that are genetically simpler than the modern alternatives because they are not the result of decades of hybridisation. The flour is coarsely (stone) ground, which delays the release of sugars and therefore lowers the GL score, and it has far fewer additives than fake flours. An added advantage of sourdough is that it is made without yeast. There is also growing evidence that sourdough fermentation may break down gluten.[5] Although the gluten in modern wheat has been widely condemned as being responsible for the rise in sensitivity to wheat, ancient wheats, such as kamut or khorasan wheat, are actually anti-inflammatory, even though they contain gluten. This leads to the inevitable conclusion that something else in modern wheat must be triggering all those immune reactions. The ill effects can't be due to gluten alone. There is little or no evidence to support the extreme view that 'all grains are poison', and, as usual, the plot thickens with every new piece of research.

Moreover, some grains are healthier than others because of the type of carbohydrate they contain. Oats are best, followed by barley and rye. Whereas the GL of wheat varies widely depending on cooking time, oats are much more consistent. Whole oat flakes, rolled oats and oatmeal (which is used to make oatcakes) are all low GL.[6] (You can lower the GL of porridge by leaving it to cool before eating – if you happen to like cold porridge!) Pick rough or jumbo oatcakes as opposed to fine, as these contain more soluble fibre, which reduces the glycaemic load. Oat pancakes, made by grinding oat flakes in a coffee/seed grinder and combining with egg and milk, are another tasty option.

Fishy breakfasts

Although they have gone out of fashion, kippers (smoked herring) make a tasty and highly nutritious low-GL breakfast. Rich in protein and omega-3 fats, a single kipper and any of the bread portions in the previous table will meet all your protein and fat needs and keep you below the 10–15 GL target.

What to eat for snacks

Grazing (eating little and often) is healthier than gorging (eating one or two big meals per day) because it helps to keep your blood sugar even.[7] This makes overeating far less likely, as you will never experience between-meal hunger pangs. For this reason, I recommend a mid-morning and a late-afternoon snack. Of these two the late-afternoon snack is most important due to the resistance factor: psychologists tell us that we spend a lot of energy during the day resisting things, and that resistance is like a muscle that gets tired. If you add low blood sugar and a glass of wine to the mix, which further lower resistance, you are inevitably going to do the wrong thing in the evening and go on a binge or choose the wrong foods for dinner. By having a late-afternoon snack before you come home from work you're more likely to stick to the programme.

Each snack should be no more than 5 GLs plus some protein, so fruit combined with nuts or seeds is a good option. The fruit portions in the table below all provide 5 GLs:

Fruit	Serving size
Strawberries	1 large punnet
Plums	4
Cherries	1 small punnet
Pear	1
Grapefruit	1
Orange	1
Apple	1 small (fits into the palm of your hand)
Peach	1 small
Melon/watermelon	1 slice

Berries – such as strawberries, raspberries, blueberries and blackberries – plums and cherries are the best fruit snacks when it comes to GL value. You can lower the GL of all these fruits by eating them with half a dozen almonds or other nuts or a tablespoon of pumpkin seeds. Almonds have the highest protein-to-calories ratio of any nut apart from chestnuts. Pumpkin seeds contain even more protein, and they are also a good source of omega-3 fats, as are walnuts and pecan nuts. I often have half an apple with a few almonds, pecan nuts or walnuts. If you travel a lot, apples and almonds are easy snacks to have on the move.

Real bread (see page 130) and a protein-rich spread, such as cottage cheese, hummus, taramasalata, or almond or peanut butter, is another good snack option. Simply halve the bread servings in the table on page 130 for an indication of 5-GL portions. Hummus tastes especially good with oatcakes, or have it on rye bread or with a raw carrot. (Even a large carrot is less than 5 GLs.) As you have probably gathered, I am a big fan of oatcakes, and indeed oats in general, which are great for weight loss and controlling blood sugar.[8] However, you should avoid any products that contain added sugar. A much better option is a sugar-free, organic oatcake, made with palm fruit oil (unsaturated fat) rather than palm oil (saturated fat) – try Nairn's brand. If you like peanut butter, buy the kind with no added sugar. Or you could have sugar-free baked beans on toast.

All these snacks are 5 GLs:

- A thin slice of rye bread/two oatcakes plus ½ small tub of cottage cheese (150g).

- A thin slice of rye bread/two oatcakes plus ⅓ small tub of hummus or taramasalata (100g).

- A thin slice of rye bread/two oatcakes and peanut butter.

- Crudités (sliced pepper, cucumber, celery or small carrot) and hummus.

- Crudités and cottage cheese, hummus or taramasalata.

- A small dairy or coconut yoghurt with no added sugar (150g), plus berries.

If you would prefer something hot, a satisfying bowl of Chestnut and Butter Bean Soup (page 164) is just 4 GLs.

As you can see, you won't be bored between meals, as there's plenty of scope for mixing and matching.

What to eat for lunch and dinner

As you will see in the next chapter, there's a host of delicious recipes that you can make for lunch and dinner, and there are even more in my *Low-GL Diet Cookbook*.

As we saw on page 122, half your plate will consist of very low-GL vegetables, such as peas, broccoli, carrots, runner beans, courgettes and kale, among many others (see pages 141–142 for the complete list). Remember, you are aiming for a total of 15 GLs for lifestyle and 10 GLs for weight loss during lunch or dinner, so this half plate of vegetables should not exceed about 3 or 4 GLs. The protein-rich quadrant might include a portion of meat, fish or tofu, while the carb-rich sector, with an allowance of 7 or 12 GLs (weight loss/lifestyle), is the place for starchier vegetables, such as parsnips or swedes, and/or grain products, such as rice, bulgur, pasta or potatoes. The 3 GLs from the vegetables, plus 7–12 GLs from the starchy carbs, adds up to 10–15 GLs, your meal allowance.

Get enough protein, but not too much

In practical terms, if you aim for 15g of protein three times a day, or 25g twice a day, you'll have enough. If you're going for an oat and not an egg breakfast, aim to eat a 10g protein breakfast and two 15 to 20g protein meals. Because the veg you eat, such as broccoli, will give you up to 5g of protein, a 15g portion of the protein food will suffice. Protein foods, such as meat, fish and eggs, are not pure protein, but also contain fat and water, so visually this looks like a quarter of what's on your plate.

More fish, less meat

It bears repeating that seafood is a rich source of omega-3 fats, which have proven health benefits, so it is a good idea to get more of your daily protein requirements from fish as well as vegetarian sources of protein, rather than meat (and especially non-organic, red or processed meat), choosing organic, grass-fed or free-range meat in preference.

How much is 15g of protein?

All the portions in the following table equate to 15g of protein. Don't eat more than three of these a day unless you're an endurance or strength athlete.

Food	Weight	Serving
Tofu and tempeh	160g	¾ packet
Soya mince	100g	3 tbsp
Chicken (with skin)	50g	1 very small breast or thigh
Turkey	50g	½ small breast

Food	Weight	Serving
Steak (rib-eye)	100g	1 small steak
Quorn	120g	⅓ pack
Salmon and trout	55g	1 very small fillet
Tuna (canned in brine)	50g	¼ can
Sardines (canned in brine)	75g	⅔ can
Cod	65g	1 very small fillet
Clams	60g	¼ can
Prawns	85g	6 large prawns
Mackerel	85g	1 medium fillet
Kipper	75g	1 large fillet
Yoghurt (natural full fat)	285g	½ large tub
Brie	75g	1 small wedge
Cheddar cheese	63g	1 small wedge
Cottage cheese	120g	½ medium tub
Full fat goat's or sheep's cheese	70g	1 small wedge
Hummus	200g	1 small tub
Milk	440ml	1 large glass
Soya milk	415ml	1 large glass
Eggs (boiled)		2
Quinoa	125g	1 large serving bowl
Baked beans	310g	¾ can
Kidney beans	175g	⅓ can
Black-eye beans	175g	⅓ can
Lentils	165g	⅓ can
Nuts (mixed)	100g	½ cup

Food	Weight	Serving
Seeds (based on pumpkin)	50g	1 small packet
Peanuts	50g	½ cup

Starchy vegetables

The carb-rich quadrant will usually be about the same size and/or weight as the protein sector, but there can be some variations; for example, if you are eating chicken with rice, the rice portion will look significantly larger than the fillet of chicken because chicken is dense and heavy whereas rice is relatively light.

Remember, this quarter of the plate should account for a maximum of 7 GLs for weight loss or 12 GLs for lifestyle, so let's see what that means in terms of portion size:

Starchy vegetables

Food	Serving size	
	7 GLs (weight loss)	12 GLs (lifestyle)
Wholegrain bulgur	Large serving, 190g	Very large serving, 325g
Pumpkin/squash	Large serving, 185g	Very large serving 320g
Carrot	160g	2 small, 270g
Swede	Large serving, 150g	Very large serving, 255g

Food	Serving size	
	7 GLs (weight loss)	12 GLs (lifestyle)
Quinoa	Large serving, 130g	Very large serving, 220g
Beetroot	Medium serving, 110g	Large serving, 190g
Cornmeal	Medium serving, 115g	Large serving, 200g
Pearl barley	Small serving, 95g	Serving, 160g
Wholemeal pasta	½ serving, 85g cooked weight	Small serving, 145g
White pasta	⅓ serving, 65g cooked weight	Small serving, 110g
Brown rice	Small serving, 70g cooked weight	Serving, 120g
White rice	⅓ serving, 45g cooked weight	½ serving, 75g
Couscous	⅓ serving, 45g soaked weight	½ serving, 75g
Broad beans	Small serving, 30g	Serving, 50g
Corn on the cob	½ cob, 60g	Small cob, 100g
Boiled potato	3 small, 75g	5 small or 3 medium,130g
Baked potato	½, 60g	1 small or ½ large, 100g
French fries	Tiny portion, 45g	Small portion, 75g
Sweet potato	½, 60g	1 small, 100g

As you can see, there are some high and some low 'value' foods on this list. The stated portions of wholegrain bulgur (which takes only eight minutes to cook) and quinoa (which takes 15 minutes) will certainly fill you up. Bulgur is delicious on its own, whereas the quinoa ideally needs some sort of flavouring, but it is a very good source of protein. Wholemeal pasta and brown rice are both much better options than the white alternatives; however, they are still quite high GL so don't go overboard on the portion size. Similarly, swedes, carrots and squashes are all preferable to potatoes. And boiled potato is better than baked potato, which is better than French fries. In reality, if you make the right choices, you'll be eating to satisfaction.

Beans and lentils

It's telling that many of the world's fattest nations have shunned beans and lentils over the past hundred years or so. They are missing out, because these are the best foods for balancing your blood sugar and providing the perfect combination of protein and carbohydrate. It's mostly due to this rare double-whammy that they have such low GL scores. Moreover, soya keeps your arteries healthy by lowering the level of 'bad' LDL cholesterol: just one serving a day, as either soya milk or tofu, can result in a 10 per cent reduction.

The portion sizes of beans and lentils can be quite generous because you are getting both protein and carbohydrate from a single food source; however, if one of these foods is the meal's primary source of protein, combine it with half the usual portion of carb-rich food; for example, if you make a lentil casserole for two people, use 200g of uncooked lentils and only 100g of uncooked brown rice. Of course, you need to do this because you are getting quite a lots of carbs – as well as protein – from the lentils.

All of the portions in the table overleaf provide the full 7 GLs for weight loss or 12 GLs for lifestyle allowance for the carb-rich sector of the plate, so you will need to reduce the quantity if you have some starchy vegetables, too. Obviously you do not need to eat the full amount given – this simply indicates the allowance. (A can of beans contains 225–245g of beans, and 200g of canned beans is roughly equivalent to 40g of dried beans.)

Legumes (peas, beans and lentils)

Food	Serving size	
	7 GLs (weight loss)	12 GLs (lifestyle)
Soya beans	4 cans	7 cans
Pinto/borlotti beans	1 can	1½ cans
Lentils	¾ can	1⅓ cans
Baked beans	¾ can	1⅓ cans
Butter beans	¾ can	1⅓ cans
Split peas	¾ can	1⅓ cans
Kidney beans	⅔ can	1 can
Chickpeas	½ can	¾ can

If you are not vegetarian, you might be quite unfamiliar with beans and lentils. Although most people have encountered dhal, baked beans, hummus and/or cassoulet, many have never thrown a packet or a tin of lentils or beans into their shopping basket. But these are immensely satisfying, flavourful foods that feature prominently in all of the world's great cuisines. They are also the main ingredients in countless mouth-watering dishes that you will find in the next chapter, from Trout with Puy Lentils and Roasted Tomatoes on the Vine (page 170) to

Borlotti Bolognese (page 165) and Chestnut and Butter Bean Soup (page 164).

Non-starchy vegetables

Now it is time to move on to the other half of the lunch or dinner plate, where you'll find the 'unlimited vegetables'. Of course, there are *some* limits, but even a generous portion of any of these foods will amount to less than 2 GL; for example, you could have a handful of peas as part of your meal.

I have listed some of the vast range of options below, with the best all-rounders in bold because these pack the biggest polyphenol/antioxidant/sirtuin-activator punch, which helps trigger autophagy, a critical part of the 5-Day Diet, and they have great benefits as part of the lifestyle diet to follow.

To recap, in general, you'll be eating two servings of non-starchy vegetables (half a plate), one serving of starchy foods and one serving of protein-rich food for both lunch and dinner. If you stick to these proportions, you will feel full at the end of every meal and may well make it all the way through to the next one without ever feeling hungry. And if hunger does strike, you can always treat yourself to a healthy snack, especially in the late afternoon.

Non-starchy vegetables

Artichokes	Brussels sprouts	Endive
Asparagus	**Cabbage**	Fennel
Aubergine	Cauliflower	Garlic
Avocado	Celery	Green beans
Beansprouts	Courgette	**Kale**
Broccoli	Cucumber	Lettuce

Mangetouts	Peppers	Spinach
Mushrooms	Radish	Spring onions
Onion	Runner beans	Tomato
Peas	Rocket	Watercress

Top tips to lower your daily GL

- Add lemon juice to meals.
- Liquidise solid food to make soup, as this is more filling.
- Soak oats or eat them as porridge.
- Chew each mouthful at least 20 times and sip water throughout the meal.
- Put your fork down on the plate between mouthfuls.
- Add a spoonful of oat bran or chia to your cereal.
- Never add sweet sauces – Dijon mustard is sugar-free and anti-inflammatory.
- Wait 30 minutes before eating something sweet.
- Save your dessert until it's time for a snack, and include some protein.

The vegetarian option

If you are a strict vegetarian, you will need to eat more beans, lentils, soya products (such as tofu and tempeh) and Quorn than either meat eaters or pescatarians (those who eat vegetarian and fish) to achieve the desired protein intake target (see the chart on pages 135–137). A serving size of tofu for a main meal is 160g – roughly three-quarters of a packet. Any meat recipes in the next chapter can be adapted by using tofu instead, and a number of recipes feature beans and lentils. I am currently working on a cookbook for vegans, applying low-GL principles.

Eat healthy fats within limits

The low-GL diet is not low fat as such, so you don't have to buy into that antiquated idea that it's eating fat that makes you fat. Conversely, it's not a high-fat diet, as in the high-fat, ketogenic diet we talk about in *The Hybrid Diet*. You'll be able to eat enough food, including fatty foods, to keep you satisfied, but it is important to use the right fats in the right ways. This is because your metabolism is on the lookout for essential fats (both omega-3 and omega-6) in the same way that you'll gravitate towards fruit if you're low in vitamin C. Eating damaged or processed fats in 'fake' foods with long lists of strange chemical ingredients won't satisfy this desire, so even though such foods might taste nice in the short term, you'll keep craving fat. On the other hand, if you're eating oily fish, good-quality olive oil, avocados, walnuts, almond butter and tahini, you'll feel satisfied even though none of these foods has a GL as such.

That is why your fat intake is not specifically limited. Your natural appetite will guide you, together with the recipes, which describe the fats to include and the quantities. But if your goal is to lose weight, but not you're succeeding, and you're bingeing on nuts, seeds and other fatty foods, it would be wise to cut back; for example, having a small handful of nuts and seeds a day is a good guide.

Good fats

Your body and brain depend on omega-3 and omega-6 essential fats. Over 90 per cent of the structural fat in your brain is the omega-3 fat DHA, which is found plentifully in oily fish. A lack can lead to poor memory, increased anxiety and depression. Both omega-3 and omega-6 fats help hormone balance, therefore a lack can lead to mood swings, PMS, sugar cravings and weight gain. Your skin gets drier, and your heart and arteries suffer. This is why these fats are called 'essential'.

Omega-3s carry a host of health benefits, not least of which is their ability to boost fat-burning.

- They reduce the risk of heart disease and sudden heart attack by 50 per cent.

- They halve the risk of ever suffering from Alzheimer's disease.

- They clear up dry skin, stimulate your metabolism, boost brain function, protect your heart and strengthen your immune system.

The low-GL diet gives you exactly the right kind and amount of essential fats, not only to help you stay healthy, but also to reduce your desire to eat unhealthy fatty foods. Even if you eat oily fish, however, you still need to supplement omega-3 fish oils rich in DHA. If you're vegan this is a health essential – there are DHA supplements that derive DHA from seaweed.

Opposite you'll see the common food sources of these fats.

Fats

Fat family	Good dietary sources
Omega-3	Fish, especially salmon, mackerel, herring, tuna and sardines; chia seeds, flax seeds, pumpkin seeds and walnuts, and their oils
Omega-6	Sunflower, sesame and pumpkin seeds and their oils; also safflower oil, corn oil, soya oil, olive oil

Bad fats

The bad fats are non-essential fats (listed on packets as saturated fats, trans fats and hydrogenated fats) found in processed meat, dairy products and processed, fried and junk foods. Saturated fat from wholefoods, including free-range, healthy animals, is not bad as such. It is just not essential.

Worst of all are the trans fats and hydrogenated fats. These are the real uglies that have been processed, fried or damaged. When the molecules of essential fats are altered by food processing or frying, they set up a reaction in the body that can damage body cells. That is why crisps, biscuits, ready-meals and fried foods are so bad for you.

The low-GL diet recipes use omega-rich foods and avoid the bad fats as much as possible. There is also an in-between fat (mono-unsaturated): omega-9, of which olive oil is a particularly rich source. This is nowhere near as good for you as the essential good fats, but it is not as bad for you as the non-essential bad fats. In fact, if the quality is good, it's good for you because it also provides polyphenols (that's why it's green in colour) and some omega-6.

Fatty foods to enjoy or avoid

Enjoy The omega-3 essential fats, found in flax, chia and pumpkin seeds, walnuts and pecan nuts, and oily coldwater fish such as mackerel, herring, salmon and tuna. These keep extra weight at bay in a number of ways.

The omega-6 essential fats are found in hot-climate seeds such as sunflower and sesame, including tahini. Olive oil also provides a little.

Avoid Foods rich in bad fats such as French fries, hamburgers, deep-fried burgers or chicken nuggets, confectionery, chocolate bars, most potato and corn chips and crisps, biscuits, doughnuts, margarine, most processed mayonnaise and salad dressings.

Unfortunately, many vegetarian processed foods are also high in these hydrogenated fats. Check the label. If it states 'partially hydrogenated vegetable oils', don't buy it.

Also avoid fried, burned or browned food.

How to use healthy fats

Here are a few tips on to how to incorporate healthy fats into your diet. You'll also find them included in many of the recipes.

- If you want to make a savoury dish creamier, try adding a teaspoon of tahini or a tablespoon of coconut milk or coconut cream.

- Use either a good-quality olive oil (see Resources) or walnut oil, which is high in omega-3, for salad dressings. These oils need to be cold pressed and stored in a light-proof container, ideally in the fridge. Some brands make a health claim on the label regarding the protection of blood lipids from oxidative stress. Treat this as a guarantee of quality, because these oils must have a very high polyphenol content to make that claim. You can lightly drizzle these oils directly onto vegetables in place of butter.

- Use a small amount of butter, ghee, coconut butter or olive oil for steam-frying (explained on page 170) and sautéing. Coconut butter adds great flavour to steam-fries.

- Have nut butter, such as almond or sugar-free peanut, on an oatcake or rye bread as a snack.

- Snack on a 5-GL portion of fruit with a small handful of nuts or seeds.

- Add pumpkin seeds and other nuts to salads.

- Try the delicious Sun-dried Tomato Pesto (see page 152) containing pine nuts and olives, as a snack on oatcakes or in dishes such as wholegrain pasta.

Top tips for healthy cooking

- Ensure that all your food is as fresh and unprocessed as possible.
- Eat more raw food: be adventurous; for example, by trying raw beetroot and carrot tops in salads.
- Cook foods in their natural, whole state, then slice or blend before serving.

▶

- Use as little water as possible during cooking, preferably by steaming, poaching or steam-frying.
- Minimise fried food in your diet.
- Favour slower, lower-temperature cooking methods.
- Never eat overcooked, charred or burned food.

Desserts

I recommend avoiding all desserts, sweets and sweetened drinks (including fruit juice) in the first couple of weeks of the lifestyle phase if your aim is to take control of your blood sugar balance and weight. You might have achieved this, however, with the 5-Day Diet. Once this has stabilised, you can allow yourself a daily allowance of 5 GLs for drinks and desserts. This means that you should still avoid desserts when eating out, because almost all restaurant sweets and puddings are loaded with white sugar and processed fat.

If you are used to eating a lot of desserts, or if you are insulin resistant, you will probably crave something sweet at the end of every meal, but it is crucial to break this habit if you want to stop your blood sugar seesawing. Fortunately, most people find that the cravings disappear after just three days. To stop them returning, it's a good idea to limit desserts to just one a week (perhaps as a treat at the weekend) after your initial sugar-free fortnight. Alternatively, continue to avoid them altogether and eat a low-GL bar, such as Pulsin's plant-based choc-fudge KetoBar which has 8.6g of carbs but only 1 GL.

When to eat

As I mentioned at the beginning of this chapter, breakfast is the most important meal of the day, and you must ensure that it contains the requisite amount of protein. Eggs are an easy way to achieve this, but if you prefer cereal, you can always add ground seeds and milk (or almond milk). This sort of breakfast will stop you experiencing hunger pangs later in the day.

In the evening, aim to finish dinner at least two hours before you go to bed. Of course, you must also ensure that this final meal of the day is low GL, with sufficient protein. Including beans, lentils or chickpeas as your 7–12 GL carb portion will help to keep your blood sugar balanced throughout the night and will even lower the GL of your breakfast the next day.

Don't eat anything after dinner, except a low-GL dessert if you haven't had a low-GL drink or dessert during the day, and aim for a minimum of eleven hours between dinner and breakfast. You can extend this to 13 or even 18 hours, starting your day with the Hybrid Latté, if you find this comfortable, thereby including that element of the 5-Day Diet. This is better once you've achieved a stable blood sugar balance – and you'll know that you have if you don't find this hard to do. You can do this every day or a couple of times a week, whatever you choose. Ensure that you get a good night's sleep because research has shown that insufficient sleep disrupts the body's appetite hormones.[9]

Sample menus

I have devised five days of menus to help you get started on the low-GL diet. I give the GL of each dish plus the daily total, up to a maximum of 40 GL a day. Use the lifestyle portion sizes to achieve 60 GLs. This means that you have an extra 5 GLs for a drink or dessert each day. Your drink and dessert options are explained in the next chapter. Thereafter, consult my *Low-GL Diet Bible*, *Low-GL Diet Cookbook* or *Ten Secrets of 100% Health Cookbook* for some excellent, low-GL ideas. There are plenty of vegan and vegetarian options in these books.

The recipes for all these dishes are in the next chapter.

Day 1

Breakfast	Get Up & Go with CarboSlow, with milk or low-carb almond milk and berries – 8 GL.
Snack	A piece of fruit, plus 5 almonds or a dessert-spoon of pumpkin seeds – 5 GL.
Lunch	Chestnut and Butter Bean Soup with 3 oat-cakes – 8 GL.
Snack	A small, no-added-sugar, plain yoghurt (150g), plus berries, or soya berry yoghurt – 5 GL.
Dinner	Thai Lamb Red Curry – 8 GL.
Total	34 GL

Day 2

Breakfast	Oat and Chia Porridge – 10 GL.
Snack	A small serving of yesterday's Chestnut and Butter Bean Soup – 4 GL.
Lunch	Walnut and Three Bean Salad (large serving) – 6 GL.
Snack	A slice of Apple and Almond Cake – 5 GL.
Dinner	Trout with Puy Lentils and Roasted Tomatoes on the Vine – 10 GL.
Total	35 GL

Day 3

Breakfast	Yoghurt and berries with chopped almonds – 5 GL.
Snack	A thin slice of bread or two oatcakes and a quarter of a small tub of hummus (50g) – 5 GL.
Lunch	Apple and Tuna Salad (large portion) – 8 GL.
Snack	A slice of Carrot and Walnut Cake – 5 GL.
Dinner	Sticky Mustard Salmon Fillets – 10 GL.
Total	33 GL

Day 4

Breakfast	Scrambled eggs on oatcakes or pumpernickel bread – 9 GL.
Snack	Crudités (sticks of carrot, pepper, cucumber or celery) and half a tub of hummus – 5 GL.
Lunch	Beany Vegetable Soup with 3 oatcakes – 8 GL.
Snack	A piece of fruit, plus 5 almonds or a dessertspoon of pumpkin seeds – 5 GL.
Dinner	Wholegrain Pasta with Borlotti Bolognese – 8 GL.
Total	35 GL

Day 5

Breakfast	Low-GL Oat Granola – 8 GL.
Snack	A thin slice of rye bread or two oatcakes, plus sugar-free peanut butter – 5 GL.
Lunch	Quinoa Tabbouleh – 8 GL.
Snack	A piece of fruit, plus 5 almonds or a dessertspoon of pumpkin seeds – 5 GL.
Dinner	Garlic Chilli Prawns with Pak Choi – 10 GL
Total	36 GL

Chapter 12

Low-GL Menus, Recipes and Drinks

All the main meals in this chapter provide no more than 10 GL, while the snacks provide no more than 5 GLs. Most are adapted from recipes in *The Low-GL Diet Bible* or *The Low-GL Diet Cookbook*, which are packed with additional dishes. The *Low-GL Diet Cookbook* is a good first step to increasing your repertoire of low-GL recipes. I am deeply indebted to my wonderful kitchen wizard, Fiona McDonald Joyce, who trained at the Institute for Optimum Nutrition and knows how to devise delicious dishes that follow all the guidelines contained within this book. We have built up a library of terrific recipes over the last ten years, many of which can be prepared incredibly quickly. Others could be served at any dinner party and receive five-star ratings without the guests ever realising they were eating something super-healthy.

Breakfasts:
- Get Up & Go with CarboSlow, Low-Carb Milk and Berries (page 154)

- Oat and Chia Porridge (page 155)

- Yoghurt and Berries with Chopped Almonds (page 156)

- Scrambled Eggs on Oatcakes or Pumpernickel (page 156)

- Low-GL Oat Granola (page 156)

Snacks:
- A piece of fruit plus 5 almonds or a dessertspoon of pumpkin seeds

- A thin piece of bread/2 oatcakes and quarter of a small tub of hummus or taramasalata (50g)

- A thin piece of bread or 2 oatcakes and peanut butter

- Crudités (sticks of carrot, pepper, cucumber or celery) and hummus or taramasalata

- A small, unsweetened, plain yoghurt (150g) and berries, or soya berry yoghurt

- A slice of Carrot and Walnut Cake (page 158) or Apple and Almond Cake (page 159)

Main meals:
Salads
A substantial serving of these provides under 10 GL. Or have half a portion as a 5-GL snack.

- Apple and Tuna Salad (page 161)

- Walnut and Three Bean Salad (page 161)

- Quinoa Tabbouleh (page 162)

Soups
- Have a big bowl (300–350g) of vegetable or bean soup. Serve with 2 or 3 rough oatcakes.

- Beany Vegetable Soup (page 163)

- Chestnut and Butter Bean Soup (page 164)

Other main meals
- Wholegrain Pasta with Borlotti Bolognese (page 165)

- Thai Lamb Red Curry (page 166)

- Garlic Chilli Prawns with Pak Choi (page 167)

- Sticky Mustard Salmon Fillets (page 168)

- Trout with Puy Lentils and Roasted Tomatoes on the Vine (page 170)

The recipes

Breakfasts

Get Up & Go with CarboSlow, Low-Carb Milk and Berries

Serves 1
1 tbsp Get Up & Go with CarboSlow

480ml unsweetened soya or almond milk, or full-fat cow's milk
a handful of blueberries, strawberries or raspberries

Blitz all the ingredients in a blender or food processor and serve.

Tip Add a teaspoon of chia seeds for extra protein, omega-3s and fibre. Make the shake watery, not too thick, and consume immediately after making. The glucomannan in CarboSlow absorbs liquid rapidly, and ideally this should happen inside you, as it will keep you feeling full for longer.

6 GL/4g carbs

Oat and Chia Porridge

Serves 1
25g oats
120ml oat, almond or soya milk
2 tsp chia seeds
a handful of berries

Simmer the oats in the milk and 120ml water for 5–10 minutes, then add the other ingredients. Stir well and serve.

Tip Half a chopped or grated apple may be used instead of the berries, and/or chopped almonds, pecan nuts or walnuts instead of the chia seeds. Add ½ teaspoon xylitol (0.5 GL) if you like.

10 GL/21g carbs

Yoghurt and Berries with Chopped Almonds

Serves 1
100g unsweetened natural sheep's, goat's, coconut or soya yoghurt
a handful of blueberries, strawberries or raspberries
a small handful of chopped or flaked almonds

Fold the yoghurt and berries together in a serving bowl, then sprinkle the almonds on top. Serve.

5 GL/25g carbs

Scrambled Eggs on Oatcakes or Pumpernickel

Serves 1
2 large eggs, beaten
2 or 3 rough oatcakes or a thin slice of pumpernickel

Cook the eggs in a small saucepan over a medium-low heat, stirring constantly with a wooden spoon, until the mixture scrambles to your preferred consistency. Serve with the oatcakes.

Tip A 25g slice of salmon may be added to the eggs. The eggs may be poached or boiled (but not fried), rather than scrambled, if you prefer.

9 GL/14g carbs

Low-GL Oat Granola

Serves 1
20g oats

20g Lizi's Low GL Granola (available in supermarkets)
240ml unsweetened oat, soya or full-fat cow's milk
2 tsp chia or pumpkin seeds
a small handful of berries

Mix the ingredients together in a serving bowl. Leave for 10 minutes or overnight, if you like. Serve.

Tip If you can't find the granola, you can just use oats instead. If not sweet enough, sprinkle with ½ teaspoon xylitol.

8 GL/20g carbs

Snacks

Sun-dried Tomato and Black Olive Pesto

The intensely savoury flavours of sun-dried tomatoes and olives make this pesto a natural with chopped fresh vegetables for a quick, substantial salad.

Serves 2 (makes 2 tablespoons of pesto)
50g sun-dried tomato paste (available in jars or tubes from supermarkets)
50g black olives, pitted
50g pine nuts
10g flat leaf parsley leaves
25g basil leaves
2 garlic cloves, crushed
1 dessertspoon lemon juice
1 tbsp olive oil
Freshly ground black pepper

1. Place all of the ingredients in a small food processor or mini chopper and blend until fairly smooth.

Tip Serve with 40g wholemeal pasta or spaghetti (dry weight) and salad (total GLs = 10) or as a snack with two oatcakes.

In the 'maintenance' phase double up the pesto quantities (to make 2 tablespoons per person) and serve with 55g wholemeal pasta or spaghetti (dry weight) and salad (total GLs = 14)

2 GL/3g carbs per serving (tablespoon)

Carrot and Walnut Cake

You can enjoy this fabulous teatime treat without feeling guilty. The walnuts, carrots and eggs all help to lower the GL score and provide plenty of nutrients. A slice is also delicious with a cup of peppermint tea at the end of a long day. If you use the walnut topping, the cake will keep well in an airtight tin for two days. If you opt for the cream cheese frosting, cover the cake and store it in the fridge. Again, it will keep for two days.

Serves 4
50g coconut oil or butter (at room temperature), plus extra
for greasing
50g xylitol
50g organic soya flour
¼ tsp baking powder
50g walnuts, ground using a blender or food processor
50g walnuts, chopped, plus 2 tbsp chopped walnuts for sprinkling
1 carrot, finely grated
2 eggs

Frosting (optional):
50g cream cheese
½ tsp vanilla extract
1 tsp xylitol

1. Preheat the oven to 180°C (160°C fan oven) Gas 4. Grease and line a 10cm cake tin with baking paper. Cream the coconut oil and xylitol together in a bowl until soft and smooth.

2. Stir in the soya flour, baking powder and ground walnuts until the mixture resembles breadcrumbs.

3. Mix in the 50g chopped walnuts and the carrot, then stir in the eggs, without beating them.

4. Spoon into the prepared cake tin and sprinkle the 2 tbsp chopped walnuts on top. Bake for 35 minutes or until the top has risen and the colour is golden. Cover the top with foil, then bake for a further 20 minutes or until the cake is fully cooked. (A skewer inserted into the centre should come out fairly clean; if the mixture is still runny, cook it for a little longer.) Leave to cool in the tin then turn out onto a cooling rack.

5. To make the frosting, if using, mix all the ingredients together in a bowl. Spread evenly over the cold cake.

5 GL/12g carbs

Apple and Almond Cake

This recipe is a healthy take on Dorset apple cake (which is full of butter and sugar). Our version provides all the taste and texture of the original, but without the gluten, sugar or dairy. It also provides plenty of fibre and minerals. It will keep well in an airtight tin for up to two days.

Serves 4
50g coconut oil or butter (at room temperature), plus extra for greasing
50g xylitol
50g organic soya flour
½ tsp baking powder
50g ground almonds
50g flaked almonds, plus 1 tbsp for sprinkling
150g Bramley apples (cored weight), unpeeled and diced
2 eggs

1. Preheat the oven to 180°C (160°C fan oven) Gas 4. Grease and line a 10cm cake tin with baking paper. Alternatively, you could use two medium-sized muffin tins, lined with paper liners.

2. Cream the coconut oil and xylitol together in a bowl until soft and smooth.

3. Stir in the flour, baking powder and ground almonds until the mixture resembles breadcrumbs.

4. Mix in the 50g flaked almonds and the apples, then stir in the eggs, without beating them.

5. Spoon into the cake tin and sprinkle the rest of the flaked almonds on top. Bake for 25 minutes or until the top is golden and set.

6. Remove from the oven and cover the top with a sheet of foil, then return to the oven for a further 20 minutes or

until the cake is fully cooked. (A skewer inserted into the centre should come out fairly clean; if the mixture is still runny, cook it for a little longer.) Leave to cool in the tin then turn out onto a cooling rack.

5 GL/4g carbs

Main meals

Apple and Tuna Salad

Serves 2
175g tin of tuna in brine, drained
1 apple, chopped
1 celery stick, sliced
1 Little Gem lettuce, torn into bite-sized pieces
1 tbsp tahini
85g natural yoghurt
2 tsp lemon juice
a pinch of sea salt
ground black pepper

Mix the tuna with the remaining ingredients. Serve.

6 GL/13g carbs

Walnut and Three Bean Salad

Serves 2
400g can mixed beans, such as haricot beans, chickpeas and flageolet beans, drained and rinsed
a handful of walnuts, roughly chopped

½ small apple, cubed
2 tsp chopped fresh flat leaf parsley or chives
1 tbsp walnut oil or olive oil
juice of 1 lemon
1 celery stick, finely chopped
a pinch of sea salt
ground black pepper
mixed salad leaves, such as spinach, rocket and watercress, to serve

Combine all the ingredients and serve with the salad leaves.

3 GL/7g carbs

Quinoa Tabbouleh

This uses quinoa in place of the traditional wholegrain bulgur,
as it is higher in protein and will keep you fuller for longer.

Serves 2
140g quinoa
280ml vegetable bouillon
1 cucumber, sliced lengthways into quarters, then finely sliced
horizontally
2 good handfuls of cherry tomatoes, chopped to the same size
as the cucumber
4 spring onions, finely sliced
a large handful of fresh mint, finely chopped
a large handful of flat leaf parsley, finely chopped
1–2 tbsp olive oil, to taste
1 tbsp lemon juice
2 tsp balsamic vinegar, or to taste

a pinch of sea salt
ground black pepper

1. Bring the quinoa to the boil in a saucepan with the bouillon, then cover, reduce the heat and simmer for 10–15 minutes until the liquid is fully absorbed and the grains are fluffy. Put the cooked quinoa in a bowl and leave it to cool.

2. When the quinoa reaches room temperature, mix in the chopped vegetables and herbs, then add the oil, lemon juice and vinegar. Season to taste.

3. Put in the fridge for at least 1 hour to allow the flavours to develop. Serve.

8 GL/15g carbs

Beany Vegetable Soup

This simple soup takes just 30 minutes to prepare from start to finish. It is also full of fibre, so it will keep you feeling satisfied for longer.

Serves 6
2 onions, chopped
3 celery sticks, finely chopped
3 leeks, sliced
450g mixed root vegetables, such as carrot, swede and parsnip, chopped into bite-sized chunks
850ml vegetable bouillon or stock
2 × 400g cans mixed pulses (such as kidney, borlotti, butter or flageolet beans or chickpeas), drained and rinsed

2 tbsp flat leaf parsley, roughly chopped
a pinch of sea salt
ground black pepper

1. Put the onions, celery, leeks, root vegetables, stock and seasoning in a large saucepan and stir. Cover and bring to the boil, then reduce the heat and simmer for 20 minutes.

2. Stir in the mixed pulses, then cover and simmer for 5–10 minutes until the vegetables and pulses are tender. Add the parsley and adjust the seasoning to taste. Serve.

8 GL/20g carbs

Chestnut and Butter Bean Soup

You can use ready-cooked chestnuts (available in larger supermarkets) to save time and effort.

Serves 4
200g cooked and peeled chestnuts (use vacuum-packed or canned to save time)
400g can butter beans, drained and rinsed
1 onion, chopped
1 carrot, chopped
2 sprigs of thyme
1.2 litres vegetable bouillon or stock
ground black pepper

1. Put all the ingredients in a large saucepan and bring to the boil. Cover, reduce the heat and simmer very gently for 35 minutes.

2. Remove from the heat and purée using a blender or food processor until smooth. Reheat if necessary and serve.

4 GL/5g carbs

Wholegrain Pasta with Borlotti Bolognese

Wholegrain pasta is now widely available as well as other high fibre/high protein alternatives, such as black bean, green lentil or chickpea pasta. Equally, you could use quinoa or spiralised ribbons of courgette.

Serves 2
1 tbsp olive oil, plus a drop for the pasta
1 onion, chopped
2 garlic cloves, crushed
1 tsp dried mixed herbs
115g button mushrooms, sliced
1 tsp vegetable bouillon powder
1 tbsp tomato purée
140g canned tomatoes
400g can borlotti beans, drained and rinsed
80g wholemeal spaghetti or penne
a pinch of salt
ground black pepper

1. Heat the oil in a saucepan and cook the onion, garlic and herbs for 2 minutes, then add the mushrooms and cook until soft.

2. Add the vegetable bouillon powder, tomato purée, tomatoes and beans, season, then simmer for 15 minutes.

3. Meanwhile, bring a saucepan of water to the boil and add the pasta. Add a drop of olive oil to the water to stop the pasta sticking. Return to the boil, then reduce the heat and simmer for 8 minutes or until tender, or as directed on the packet.

4. Drain the pasta in a colander. Serve the pasta with the Bolognese on top.

10 GL/22g carbs

Thai Lamb Red Curry

If you like a bit of extra heat in your curry, you can always add some fresh red chillies.

Serves 4
1 tbsp coconut oil or virgin rapeseed oil
4 tsp Thai red curry paste
450g lamb leg, diced
50g unsalted cashew nuts, blitzed in a food processor
1 tbsp tomato purée
400ml full-fat coconut milk
2 kaffir lime leaves, roughly crumbled
200g wholegrain bulgur
150g mangetouts or fine green beans
1 tbsp fish sauce
lime wedges, to serve

1. Heat the oil in a wok over a high heat. Stir-fry the curry paste for 1 minute, then add the lamb and stir-fry to coat it in the paste.

2. Tip in the cashew nuts, tomato purée, coconut milk and lime leaves and bring to the boil.

3. Reduce the heat slightly, then cover and simmer, stirring occasionally, for 50–60 minutes until the sauce has reduced and thickened.

4. After about 45 minutes, bring a saucepan of water to the boil and cook the wholegrain bulgur for 8 minutes.

5. Shortly before serving, boil or steam the mangetouts until al dente, then stir them into the curry along with the fish sauce.

6. Serve the curry with the wholegrain bulgur and squeeze over the juice from the lime wedges.

8 GL/12g carbs

Garlic Chilli Prawns with Pak Choi

A simple marinade adds a lot of flavour to the prawns to make this a tasty and satisfying meal. You can simply add chilli flakes to normal oil if you are unable to find chilli-infused oil.

Serves 2
3 garlic cloves, crushed
juice of 2 limes
1 green chilli, deseeded
1 tsp chilli-infused oil (or dried chilli flakes in olive oil)
a large pinch of sea salt
4 tbsp virgin rapeseed oil
300g large fresh, raw prawns, fully prepared

100g wholegrain bulgur or 80g quinoa
250g pak choi, stems separated from the leaves, and both stems and leaves roughly chopped
1 tbsp oyster sauce

1. Blend the garlic, lime, chilli, chilli oil, salt and 3 tbsp of the rapeseed oil to a purée using a blender. Put this mixture into a shallow bowl and add the prawns. Stir to coat well. Leave to marinate for 20 minutes at room temperature.

2. Bring a pan of water to the boil and cook the wholegrain bulgur for 8 minutes (or the quinoa for 10–15 minutes) until tender. Drain in a sieve.

3. Heat a griddle pan or frying pan until medium hot, then cook the prawns for 1½ minutes each side.

4. Heat the remaining 1 tbsp rapeseed oil in a wok or frying pan over a medium-high heat and stir-fry the pak choi stems for 1 minute, then add the leaves and cook for 3 minutes more.

5. Remove the wok from the heat and stir in the oyster sauce. Serve immediately with the prawns and the wholegrain bulgur (or quinoa).

10 GL/18g carbs

Sticky Mustard Salmon Fillets

This dish requires a bit of planning as you need to allow enough time to marinate the fillets before cooking them; however, thereafter, they are simply baked, which gives you plenty of time to prepare everything else, so this is a great option when you have people over for dinner.

Serves 2
juice and grated zest of ½ orange
1 tsp wholegrain mustard
1 tsp clear honey
2 small skinless, boneless salmon fillets
100g wholegrain bulgur or 80g quinoa, or 3 baby new potatoes
a large bunch of spinach
1 or 2 red or yellow peppers, deseeded and chopped

1. Whisk the orange juice and zest into the mustard and honey in a small bowl.

2. Put the salmon fillets in a shallow ovenproof dish and pour over the orange mixture. Leave to marinate for 30–60 minutes in the fridge. Meanwhile, preheat the oven to 180°C (160°C fan oven) Gas 4.

3. Bake the salmon for 20–25 minutes.

4. Meanwhile, bring a saucepan of water to the boil and cook the wholegrain bulgur for 8 minutes (or the quinoa or potatoes for 10–15 minutes) until tender.

5. Five minutes before serving, steam or steam-fry (see box on page 170) the spinach and peppers. Serve with the bulgur and salmon.

10 GL/17g carbs

Steam-frying

Steam-frying is a good way to cook vegetables, because it adds lots of flavour and it doesn't destroy nutrients in the same way that frying does.

To steam-fry, use a shallow pan or a deep frying pan with a thick base and a lid that seals well. You can steam-fry without oil by first adding 2 tablespoons of liquid to the pan – water, vegetable stock, soy sauce or a little watered-down sauce that you are going to use for the dish. Add your vegetables and cook rapidly for 1–2 minutes, then turn up the heat, add 1–2 tablespoons more of the liquid and clamp the lid on tightly. After 1 minute, add the remaining ingredients. Turn the heat down after a couple of minutes and steam in this way until cooked.

Alternatively, add 1 teaspoon–1 tablespoon olive oil, butter or coconut oil to the pan, warm it, add the ingredients and cook. After 2 minutes, add 3 tablespoons of liquid as above and clamp on the lid. Steam the ingredients until done.

Trout with Puy Lentils and Roasted Tomatoes on the Vine

Serves 2
85g Puy lentils
1 tsp vegetable bouillon powder
1 tsp mixed dried herbs
2 small trout fillets

12 cherry tomatoes on the vine
ground black pepper
2 slices of lemon and a handful of fresh flat leaf parsley,
chopped, to garnish

1. Preheat the oven to 190°C (170°C fan oven) Gas 5. Put the
    lentils in a saucepan and add water to cover. Bring to the
    boil, then reduce the heat and simmer for 20 minutes or until
    the water is almost absorbed. The lentils should be soft to the
    bite, but don't worry if they seem a little hard – Puy lentils
    retain their shape and have a satisfyingly chewy texture
    when cooked. Add the bouillon powder and mixed herbs.

2. Put the fish in a non-stick roasting tin and lay the
    tomatoes around them, then bake for 12–15 minutes or
    until cooked through.

3. Serve the lentils with the trout and tomatoes, sprinkled
    with black pepper and garnished with the lemon
    and parsley.

10 GL/14g carbs

What to drink

The best drink for both general health and fat burning is water.
You should aim to consume the equivalent of 2 litres, or eight
glasses, each day. If this seems an enormous amount, bear in
mind that you can factor in tea and coffee (and juices in the
lifestyle phase).

Leaving a bottle on your desk will remind you to keep it
topped up. Like the rest of the lifestyle diet, drinking plenty of

fluid will eventually become second nature, and it will leave you feeling much better in every way.

Cold drinks and juices

You must avoid fruit juice during the 5-Day Diet, but it's generally best to avoid it anyway; however, during the lifestyle phase, you could drink a half-shot of Blueberry Active (made from pure blueberries) or Cherry Active (made from Montmorency cherries), because they are both low GL and very high in antioxidants. It might be worth working out a way to include this in the lifestyle phase – I often add it to my water bottle for flavour, for example.

All commercial fruit juices, whether concentrated or freshly squeezed, have a relatively high GL because the fibre has been removed. The best is probably cloudy apple juice, although even this should be drunk diluted – half juice and half water or, even better, two-thirds water to one-third juice.

The following table indicates 5-GL portions for a variety of drinks.

Non-alcoholic drinks

Drink	Serving size
Tomato juice	500ml
Carrot juice	1 small glass
Grapefruit juice, unsweetened	1 small glass
Apple juice, unsweetened	1 small glass, diluted 50:50 with water

Drink	Serving size
Orange juice, unsweetened	1 small glass, diluted 50:50 with water; or freshly squeezed juice of 1 orange
Blueberry Active	20ml (1 tbsp) of concentrate
Cherry Active	20ml (1 tbsp) of concentrate
Pineapple juice	½ small glass, diluted 50:50 with water
Cranberry juice	½ small glass, diluted 50:50 with water
Grape juice	2cm in a glass – avoid!

Stay away from all fizzy, sweetened and caffeinated drinks as well as sugar-sweetened cordials.

A good rule of thumb is to have no more than one glass of juice each day, diluting it as need be so that you never have more than 5 GLs in the course of the day. You could have either a small glass of carrot juice or a small glass of diluted apple juice – but not both! Always drink slowly – sip rather than gulp – as this helps to retard the release of the sugars in the juice (as does diluting).

Remember, you have a daily 5 GL-allowance on the weight-loss diet for drinks or desserts, so, if you do have a 5-GL drink, don't have a dessert.

Coffee

During the 5-Day Diet you'll start your day with the Hybrid Fast Latté containing coffee (or decaf if you prefer). In addition to acting as an energiser and appetite suppressant, coffee actually increases ketone levels and encourages the body to release stored fat, which the liver can then convert into more ketones. One recent study gave a group of volunteers the equivalent of either two or four cups of coffee and found that the higher dose had a greater impact on the level of ketones.[1]

Is coffee good for you? A 2014 study concluded that coffee drinkers have less risk of developing diabetes than non-coffee drinkers.[2] On the other hand, two years later, a meta-analysis of seven previous trials asserted that caffeine makes the body less sensitive to insulin, which causes blood sugar to rise: 'Acute caffeine ingestion reduces insulin sensitivity in healthy subjects. Thus, in the short term, caffeine might shift glycaemic homeostasis toward hyperglycemia,' reported the authors.[3] Another study also found that insulin sensitivity deteriorates and blood sugar level rises as caffeine dose increases.[4] This suggests that it is something else in coffee – not the caffeine – that provides protection against diabetes, especially as decaf has no impact on insulin sensitivity.

One thing is certain: coffee is much more harmful when it is drunk with a high-carb snack. A group of researchers gave volunteers a carbohydrate snack, such as a croissant, muffin or toast, together with either decaf or caffeinated coffee.[5] Those in the second group experienced far greater increases in blood sugar (on average, their levels rose three times more than those who drank decaf), and their insulin sensitivity almost halved. Drinking coffee with carbs, therefore, should be avoided at all times.

If you love your coffee, my advice is to have one in the morning, without any food, and to monitor your glucose and ketone levels (see Chapter 9). Certainly avoid it after midday, because it suppresses melatonin (which you need in order to sleep well) for up to ten hours.

Green and black tea

From every point of view, I recommend green tea rather than black tea, although the latter is not bad either; for example, green tea lowers blood glucose and improves insulin sensitivity, according to a meta-analysis of seventeen trials.[6] However, it has neither a positive nor a negative effect on people with diabetes.[7] Tea also contains theanine, a relaxing amino acid that counters the adrenalising impact of the caffeine it contains. Traditionally, the Japanese left the green tea leaves in the pot and used them to make a run-through if they wanted another drink. Such run-throughs have relatively more antioxidants and polyphenols and relatively less caffeine.

Chocolate

Cacao, the sirtuin activator in dark chocolate (sirtuin help trigger autophagy), also helps to improve insulin sensitivity[8] and lower blood sugar. Dark chocolate is also an appetite suppressant (in marked contrast to either white or milk chocolate), so it's by far the best option as long as you eat a low-GL variety.[9] In practical terms, this means that it needs to be 80 per cent cacao. If you use sugar-free cacao powder and low-GL milk (such as unsweetened soya or carb-free almond milk) to make hot chocolate, you can always sweeten it with a little xylitol. Note that I include a teaspoon of unsweetened raw cacao powder in my Hybrid Latté (see page 61).

Alcohol

You need to avoid alcohol completely during the 5-Day Diet because it will disrupt autophagy and also because your body is already detoxifying, as you burn fat, and alcohol adds to that burden.

Although pure alcohol, such as a neat shot of vodka, tequila, gin or whisky, has 0 GL and can even raise ketones, it contains calories that your body will burn in preference to fat. Moreover, the liver can convert any alcohol that is not burned for energy directly into triglycerides, which can then be converted into ketones (which is why you sometimes see an increase in ketones after drinking); however, if you are not in ketosis, this increase in triglycerides will just make you fat. This is why alcohol consumption is routinely associated with weight gain. On the other hand, if you are in ketosis and drink too much alcohol, the body will be able to meet all its energy requirements from the booze and will stop converting body fat into ketones, so go easy.

Secondly, alcohol is a toxin, so the body has to flush it out of the system, which interferes with normal, healthy metabolism. Thirdly, it contains no nutrients. Finally, and perhaps most importantly, it weakens willpower, which might leave you scoffing carbs in the evening despite your best intentions.

It will take less alcohol than usual to leave you feeling drunk during ketosis, so, for this reason alone, it's a good idea to limit yourself to a maximum of one drink per day in the high-fat phase. Moreover, if you drink any more than this, you are likely to suffer a very bad hangover.

When on the low-GL lifestyle diet, stick to those drinks that have the least carbs: dry white wine, or champagne, is better than dessert wine. Remember, you have a daily allowance of 5 GLs for all drinks and desserts so, assuming you've had no fruit juice or desserts during the day, you can allow yourself up to 5 GLs of alcohol.

As you will see from the table below, from a GL standpoint, your best options are neat spirits, then white wine, red wine and finally beer. If you are a beer drinker, limit yourself to just half a pint or a small beer every other day (or choose a low-carb beer). By contrast, if you prefer dry white wine, you can have a glass every day and still have 4 GLs left over for a dessert or a small glass of diluted apple juice. As a general rule, however, don't have more than 1 unit a day, or a maximum of 6 units a week.

Alcoholic drinks

Drink	GL	Units	Daily maximum
Beer/lager, ½ pint (330ml)	10	1	¼ pint
Red wine, small glass (115ml)	2	1	1
White wine, small glass (115ml)	1	1	1
Spirit shot (30ml)	0	1	1
Spirit and orange juice (125ml juice)	6	1	1 small
Spirit and cola (125ml cola)	8	1	1 very small

Chapter 13

Support Supplements

There are some 30 vitamins and minerals that are essential for health. Many of them, together with vitamin C, will help you to burn fat. They boost your metabolism and re-programme your body to turn food into energy rather than fat. These aren't drugs; they're nutrients, and they will help to fine-tune your metabolism as an integral part of the low-GL diet, whether for weight loss or lifestyle. I've researched the optimal level of these nutrients and it's not possible to achieve them solely with diet, but why might this be?

Throughout evolution humankind consumed more calories than today because we expended more while hunting, gathering, walking, chopping wood, fetching water – just living. We also ate more, and all the food was fresh (and, of course, organic). It was only when cars, fridges and refining came along that we didn't need to eat so much, and we could also store food; however, the level of nutrients that our ancestors needed – for example, for a healthy brain – hasn't changed, and we might even need more of some of them in order to support our mentally active modern lifestyles. Today, we need to obtain all these nutrients from substantially less food, which lacks the nutritional quantity and quality of food from the past because of the depletion of nutrients in the soil where our food is grown. When we choose refined foods this exacerbates the problem of nutrient deficiency.

Fat-burning supplements – the basics

I recommend that you supplement your well-balanced diet with fat-burning vitamins and minerals, even if you are following the lifestyle diet with no need for weight loss, to ensure your metabolism is working at peak efficiency. The chart that follows gives ideal supplement levels for an average person who is eating a healthy, balanced diet. The easiest way to take these every day is in a high-strength multivitamin and mineral, plus 1,000mg of vitamin C and an essential omega-3 supplement. (The most powerful omega-3 fats are called DHA and EPA. The most powerful omega-6 fat is called GLA. You need ten times more DHA plus EPA combined than GLA.) I take these three supplements every day in my packs, which are provided in convenient strips, taking two strips a day.

Most health-food shops can help you to find supplements to meet these levels in the simplest and least expensive way, choosing from a variety of good brands. Supplements should be taken with food, preferably with breakfast, or spread throughout the day.

Additional supplements

During the first three months of starting the low-GL lifestyle diet, whether for weight loss or long-term good health, you can help to stabilise your appetite and sugar cravings by taking, in addition to the above, a combination of the supplements HCA and chromium, plus glucomannan fibre.

I talked about HCA and chromium in Chapter 8, as these are recommended in the 5-Day Diet. In Chapter 4 I explained the role of glucomannan fibre to support your digestion, but glucomannan also promotes healthy weight loss. An evaluation by the European Food Safety Authority (EFSA) concluded that glucomannan, if taken at a daily dosage of 3 grams, can assist weight loss taken in the context of a controlled diet. This is based on a review of nine studies.[1] As an example, one study gave 20 obese volunteers either 1 gram of glucomannan fibre in two capsules, taken three times a day, or a placebo. At the end of eight weeks those on the glucomannan had lost 5.5kg (12lb), while those on the placebo had gained 1.5kg (3lb), so there was a 7kg (15lb) difference in weight loss. This amount of glucomannan is equivalent to half a teaspoon of powder, or two capsules, taken with a large glass of water before each meal.

While chromium is particularly useful if you have sugar cravings, glucomannan helps you feel fuller and is therefore good for those who don't feel full enough between meals.

These are the daily levels you need for maximum effect. For the first three months only, supplement with additional chromium, HCA and glucomannan fibre, especially if you are prone to sugar cravings and have poor appetite control.

Recommended supplement levels

Vitamins	Optimum daily intake	Health benefits
Vitamin A	1,500mcg	Immune strength
Vitamin B1 (thiamine)	25mg	Makes energy
Vitamin B2 (riboflavin)	25mg	Makes energy
Vitamin B3 (niacin)	50mg	Lowers cholesterol
Vitamin B5 (pantothenate)	50mg	Improves memory
Vitamin B6 (pyridoxine)	50mg	Balances hormones
Vitamin B12 (cobalamine)	10mcg	Vital for energy
Folic acid	200mcg	Protects your DNA
Biotin	50mcg	Makes energy
Vitamin C	1,000mg	Boosts immunity
Vitamin D	5mcg	Builds bones
Vitamin E (d-alpha tocopherol)	100mg	Protects arteries

Minerals	Optimum daily intake	Health benefits
Calcium	200mg	Builds bones
Magnesium	150mg	Keeps you relaxed
Iron	10mg	Carries oxygen
Zinc	10mg	Boosts immunity
Manganese	3mg	Metabolic support
Chromium	30mcg	Balances blood sugar

Essential fats	Optimum daily intake	Health benefits
Omega-3 (EPA + DHA)	500mg	Brain essential
Omega-6 (GLA)	50mg	Balances hormones

Supplement	Daily intake	Health benefits
Hydroxycitric acid (HCA)*	2,500mg	Turns food into energy, not fat
Chromium**	200–400mcg	Reduces sugar craving
Glucomannan fibre***	3,000mg	Supports the digestion

*One 750mg tablet three times a day, taken 15 minutes before main meals

**200mcg taken twice daily, with a mid-morning and afternoon snack.

***1,000mg taken three times daily, before meals, with a large glass of water.

As you will have bought these supplements anyway for the 5-Day Diet, there is no harm, and plenty of benefit, in continuing to take them once you finish the five days. All these supplements are easy to find in most health-food shops.

Supplement facts

If you want the best weight-loss results possible, supplements should not be seen as an optional extra but as a central part of your weight-loss and health success. My own research has shown that:

- Following the low-GL diet on its own will enable you to lose weight.

- Following the low-GL diet and taking a multivitamin and mineral with vitamin C will help you to lose more weight than the diet alone.

- Following the diet and taking the multivitamin and mineral with vitamin C and taking additional chromium and HCA supplements will lead to maximum weight loss.

This means that supplements make a positive and healthy difference to weight loss. Once you've achieved your ideal weight, you don't need to keep taking these extras.

Chapter 14

Exercise for Life

In combination with what you eat, exercise helps to stabilise your blood sugar levels and reduce your appetite – and you can achieve all this, and maintain fitness and muscle mass in just 15 minutes a day. The human body needs physical activity to work properly, just as it needs water or vitamins. One critical function, appetite control, goes wrong when you do no exercise at all. You will eat disproportionately more than you need. The right kind of exercise will increase muscle and boost the rate at which you burn fat for up to 15 hours afterwards. A pound (0.5kg) of muscle burns many more calories a day than a pound of fat; so every pound of fat you lose and every pound of muscle you gain will further increase your body's long-term ability to burn fat.

That's why any diet should always be combined with specific types of exercise, because, although cutting carbs and calories has positive health benefits (such as reducing high levels of glucose and insulin), it also puts your muscles under threat. This is because the rapid fall in carbs or calories turns off the body's fat controller – mTOR – the enzyme that is responsible for muscle growth. In search of fresh supplies of glucose, the body turns to protein, which is found in the muscles, and breaks it down into its constituent amino acids. While this is happening, the best way to preserve muscle is through exercises that maintain and renew it. This is unlikely to be a concern if you go ketogenic for five days in the 5-Day Diet phase, however, but it would be if you did it for a month.

Exercise makes it less likely that muscle tissue will be transported to the liver for recycling into glucose, because a resistance or strength workout – that is, exercises that are designed to build muscle – switches mTOR back on for a short period of time. Just eight minutes of appropriate exercise every other day is enough. The exercises can be done on gym machines or using rubber resistance bands; simple press-ups will also suffice.

Of course, when the body's mTOR is reactivated, you need sufficient protein in your diet to build muscle. Don't worry, though, I've taken this into consideration in my low-GL lifestyle diet. It is a myth that you need to eat lots of protein, and lots of meat, to make muscle. You just need enough, and vegetable protein is as good as, if not better than, animal protein. Also, remember that mTOR is switched off by caffeine, so make sure that you have your morning coffee at least 30 minutes before exercising. You'd be better off eating after exercise. This is also consistent with evolution: you hunt then eat, not the other way around.

If you do no strengthening/resistance exercises on a regular basis, you are likely to lose as much as 40 per cent of your muscle mass by the time you are eighty.[2] And you can ill afford to do that, because muscle is needed for the production of several crucial chemicals that start to decline as you get older, including human growth hormone (hGh) – which may have anti-ageing benefits – testosterone and dehydroepiandrosterone (DHEA). Muscle is also more metabolically active than fat (that is, it burns far more calories), so if you lose muscle mass, you gain more weight, despite eating the same number of calories.

You also need to supplement resistance training with aerobic exercise – brisk walking, jogging, running, dancing or cycling (in short, anything that makes your heart beat faster and gets you sweating) – as this will strengthen your heart, burn calories and help you to lose that dangerous belly fat. Aerobic exercise raises your metabolic rate for 24 hours, so you will benefit from increased fat burning for a whole day.

Interval training

Standard aerobic workouts don't do much for muscle building. What you need are short, sharp bursts of flat-out activity. At first, this might involve alternating two minutes of low-intensity walking with two minutes of brisk walking for a total of 30 minutes. Gradually, though, you might aim to build up to two minutes of walking and two minutes of jogging, then two minutes of jogging on the flat coupled with two minutes uphill, or two minutes of jogging and two minutes of hard running. Any, or all, of these can be done on a treadmill at the gym if that is more convenient.

As you get more experienced, you could sprint flat out for one minute, then switch to a gentle recovery pace for three minutes, then go flat out again; however, you will need to do this at least half a dozen times per session to see any significant muscle-building effect.

Cardio and strength training – the dynamic duo

One of the simplest and most practical ways to achieve the best of both worlds is to stick to the weekly exercise routine that was developed by the former Gladiator Kate Staples and described in 'A recommended exercise routine' on page 70.

The combination of exercise, eating a low-GL diet as your baseline, doing the 5-Day Diet four times a year and daily supplementation to provide your cells with optimum nutrition is a winning formula for adding years to your life and life to your years. Far too many people suffer too much and die too young simply because they do not understand how to give their body what it needs. I hope this book, as well as giving you a short-term 'fix', has expanded your awareness about how your body works.

Monitor Your Progress Chart

Use the following charts to see at a glance how you are getting on with your 5-Day Diet. You can photocopy them if you wish.

Your health statistics

Statistics	Initial	Final	Change
Body fat percentage			
Weight			
Hip			
Waist			
Waist:hip ratio			

Glucose and ketone measures

Day	Glucose	Ketones (blood)	Ketones (breath)	GKI (glucose/ ketones)
-1				
1				
2				
3				
4				
5				
6				

Health issues

		Week before diet (average)	Final (Day 6)	Week after diet (average)	Change
1	Energy	/10	/10	/10	
2		/10	/10	/10	
3		/10	/10	/10	

References

Introduction

1 https://www.ncbi.nlm.nih.gov/pubmed/31025151 – Provocative Question: Should Ketogenic Metabolic Therapy Become the Standard of Care for Glioblastoma?
    T.N. Seyfried, et al., *Neurochem Res.* 2019 Oct;44(10):2392–404

Chapter 1

1 J. Finnell, et al., 'Is fasting safe? A chart review of adverse events during medically supervised, water-only fasting', *BMC Complement Altern Med.* 2018 18:67 doi: 10.1186/s12906-018-2136-6

2 M. Wei, et al., 'Fasting-mimicking diet and markers/risk factors for aging, diabetes, cancer and cardiovascular disease', *Science Translational Medicine*, (2017), vol. 9 (377):pii:eaai8700

3 https://www.immunology.org/news/
    report-reveals-the-rising-rates-autoimmune-conditions

4 C. Cheng, et al., 'Fasting-mimicking diet promotes ngn3-driven β-cell regeneration to reverse diabetes' 2017, *Cell*. 168; 775–88

5 P. Rangan, et al., 'Fasting-mimicking diet modulates microbiota and promotes intestinal regeneration to reduce inflammatory bowel disease pathology, *Cell Reports*, (2019) 26, 2704–19 March 5, 2019 https://doi.org/10.1016/j.celrep.2019.02.019

6 M.A. Cooper, et al., 'A ketogenic diet reduces metabolic syndrome-induced allodynia and promotes peripheral nerve growth in mice', *Experimental Neurology* (2018) Aug.;306:149–57

7 L.S. Whyte, 'Endo-lysosomal and autophagic dysfunction: A driving

factor in Alzheimer's disease?', *Journal of Neurochemistry*, (2017), vol. 140(5):703–17

8 M. Fortier, et al., *Alzheimer's & Dementia* 2019; 1–10

9 M. Phillips, et al., 'Low-fat versus ketogenic diet in Parkinson's disease: A pilot randomized controlled trial', *Movement Disorders*, (2018); 33(8):1306–14

10 C. Craig, 'Mitoprotective dietary approaches for myalgic enceph-alomyelitis/chronic fatigue syndrome: Caloric restriction, fasting, and ketogenic diets', *Med Hypotheses*, (2015);85(5):690–3

11 M. Nei, et al., 'Ketogenic diet in adolescents and adults with epilepsy', *Seizure*, (2014);23(6):439–42

12 C. Vandenberghe, et al., 'Tricaprylin alone increases plasma ketone response more than coconut oil or other medium-chain triglycerides: An acute crossover study in healthy adults', *Current Developments in Nutrition*, (2017) vol. 1(4):e000257

Chapter 2

1 C. H. Hsieh, et al., 'Functional impairment in miro degradation and mito-phagy is a shared feature in familial and sporadic Parkinson's disease', *Cell Stem Cell*, (2016), vol. 19:709–24

2 E. White, 'Autophagy, metabolism, and cancer', *Clinical Cancer Research*, (2015), vol. 21(22):5037–46

3 N.S. Katheder, et al., 'Microenvironmental autophagy promotes tumour growth', *Nature*, (2017), vol. 541:417–20

4 V. Lahiri, 'Eat yourself to live: Autophagy's role in health and disease', *Scientist*, (2018)

5 C. Tomas, et al., 'Cellular bioenergetics is impaired in patients with chronic fatigue syndrome', *PLoS One*, (2017), vol. 12(10):e0186802

6 C. Craig, 'Mitoprotective dietary approaches for myalgic encephalo-myelitis/chronic fatigue syndrome: Caloric restriction, fasting, and ketogenic diets', *Medical Hypotheses*, (2015), vol. 85(5):690–3

7 M.H. Hoang, et al., 'Kaempferol reduces hepatic triglyceride accumulation by inhibiting Akt', *Journal of Food Biochemistry*, (2019) Sept. 5:e13034. doi: 10.1111/jfbc.13034

8 H. Gu, et al., 'Nicotinate-curcumin impedes foam cell formation from THP-1 cells through restoring autophagy flux', *Public Library of Sciences One*, (2016) Apr. 29;11(4):e0154820; see also H. Gu, et al., 'Nicotinate-curcumin ameliorates cognitive impairment in diabetic rats by rescuing autophagic flux in CA1 hippocampus', *CNS Neuroscience and Therapeutics*,

(2019) Apr.;25(4):430–41; see also C.S. Wu, et al., 'Curcumin functions as a MEK inhibitor to induce a synthetic lethal effect on KRAS mutant colorectal cancer cells receiving targeted drug regorafenib', *Journal of Nutritional Biochemistry*, (2019) Aug. 31;74:108227

9 M. Arlorio, et al., 'Protective activity of Theobroma cacao L. phenolic extract on AML12 and MLP29 liver cells by preventing apoptosis and inducing autophagy', *Journal of Agricultural and Food Chemistry*, (2009) Nov. 25;57(22):10612–8. doi: 10.1021/jf902419t

10 J. Chung, et al., 'Trans-cinnamic aldehyde inhibits aggregatibacter actinomycetemcomitans-induced inflammation in THP-1-derived macrophages via autophagy activation', *Journal of Peridontology*, (2018) Oct;89(10):1262–1271. doi: 10.1002/JPER.17–0727. Epub 2018 Aug. 30

11 F.Pietrocola, et al., 'Calorie restriction mimetics enhance anticancer immunosurveillance' 2016, *Cancer Cell* Jull 11:30(1):147-160

12 M. Karim, et al., 'Effect and proposed mechanism of vitamin C modulating amino acid regulation of autophagic proteolysis', *Biochimie*, 2017 Nov.;142:51–62

13 A. Martin, et al., 'Stimulatory effect of vitamin C on autophagy in glial cells', *Journal of Neurochemistry*, (2002);82(3):538–49

14 Y. Zhang, et al., 'DHA supplementation improves cognitive function via enhancing Aβ-mediated autophagy in Chinese elderly with mild cognitive impairment: A randomised placebo-controlled trial', *Journal of Neurology, Neurosurgery and Psychiatry*, (2018);89(4):382–8

15 https://health.gov/dietaryguidelines/dga2005/report/HTML/table_g2_adda2.htm

Chapter 4

1 H.L. Chen, et al., 'Supplementation of konjac glucomannan into a low-fibre Chinese diet promoted bowel movement and improved colonic ecology in constipated adults: A placebo-controlled, diet-controlled trial', *Journal of the American College of Nutrition*, (2008) Feb;27(1):102–8

Chapter 5

1 L. Hou, et al., 'Essential role of autophagy in fucoxanthin-induced cytotoxicity to human epithelial cervical cancer HeLa cells', *Acta Pharmacol Sin*, 2013 Nov.;34(11):1403–10

Chapter 8

1   S. Davies, 'Zinc, nutrition & health' chapter in J. Bland, 1984/5, *Yearbook of Nutritional Medicine*, Keats, 1985

2   R. Chen, et al., 'Study on the protective mechanism of autophagy on cartilage by magnesium sulfate' (2018) Oct 15;32(10):1340–5

3   See https://www.epsomsaltcouncil.org/wp-content/uploads/2015/10/report_on_absorption_of_magnesium_sulfate.pdf

4   S.L. Pinkosky, et al., 'Targeting ATP-citrate lyase in hyperlipidemia and metabolic disorders', *Trends in Molecular Medicine* (2017), vol. 23(11), pp. 1047–63

5   N. Han, et al., '(-)-hydroxycitric acid nourishes protein synthesis via altering metabolic directions of amino acids in male rats', *Phytotherapy Research* (2016), vol. 30(8), pp. 1316–29

6   R. Sripradha and S.G. Magadi, 'Efficacy of *Garcinia Cambogia* on body weight, inflammation and glucose tolerance in high fat fed male wistar rats', *Journal of Clinical and Diagnostic Research* (2015), vol. 9(2): BF01–BF0

7   I. Onakpoya et al, 'The use of *garcinia* extract (hydroxycitric acid) as a weight loss supplement: A systematic review and meta-analysis of randomised clinical trials', *Journal of Obesity* (2011), vol. 2011:509038

8   H. Preuss, et al., 'An overview of the safety and efficacy of a novel, natural hydroxycitric acid extract (HCA-SX) for weight management', *Journal of Medicine* (2004), vol. 35(1–6), pp. 33–48

9   L.O. Chuah, et al., 'In vitro and in vivo toxity of garcinia or hydroxycitric acid: A review', *Evidence-Based Complementary and Alternative Medicine* (2012), vol. 2012:197920

10 S. Davies, et al., 'Age-related decreases in chromium levels in 51,665 hair, sweat and serum samples from 40,872 patients: Implications for the prevention of cardiovascular disease and type II diabetes mellitus', *Metabolism* (1997), vol. 46(5), pp. 1–4

11 Y.L. Chen, et al., 'The effect of chromium on inflammatory markers, 1st and 2nd phase insulin secretion in type 2 diabetes', *European Journal of Nutrition*, vol. 53(1), pp. 127–33. See also Drake T, Endo, Pract, 2012

12 S. Anton, 'Effects of chromium picolinate on food intake and satiety', *Diabetes Technology & Therapeutics* (2008), vol. 10(5), pp. 405–12

13 K.A. Brownley, et al., 'Chromium supplementation for menstrual cycle-related mood symptoms', *Journal of Dietary Supplements* (2013), vol. 10(4), pp. 345–56

14 J.R. Davidson, et al., 'Effectiveness of chromium in atypical depression: A placebo-controlled trial', *Biological Psychiatry* (2003), vol. 53(3), pp. 261–4. See also K.A. Brownley, et al., 'A double-blind, randomized pilot trial of

chromium picolinate for binge eating disorder', *Journal of Psychosomatic Research* (2013), vol. 75(1), pp. 36–72

15 N. Cheng, et al., 'Follow-up survey of people in China with type-2 diabetes consuming supplemental chromium', *Journal of Trace Elements in Experimental Medicine* (1999), vol. 12(2), pp. 55–60

16 N. Suksomboon, et al., 'Systematic review and meta-analysis of the efficacy and safety of chromium supplementation in diabetes', *Journal of Clinical Pharmacy and Therapeutics* (2014), vol. 39(3), pp. 292–306

Chapter 11

1 C. Hopkins et al., *Sleep* (2017), vol. 40(S1), http://www.sleepmeeting.org/docs/default-source/attendee-documents/abstractbook2017.pdf?sfvrsn=2

2 S. Wehrens, et al., 'Meal timing regulates the human circadian system', *Current Biology* (2017), vol. 27(12):1768–75. See also L. Ruddick-Collins, et al., 'The Big Breakfast Study: Chrono-nutrition influence on energy expenditure and bodyweight', *Nutrition Bulletin* (2018), vol. .43(2):174–83; C. Hopkins, et al., 'Delayed eating adversely impacts weight and metabolism compared with daytime eating in normal weight adults', *Sleep* (2017), vol. 40(S1): 24

3 J. Warren, et al., 'Low glycaemic index breakfasts and reduced food intake in preadolescent children', *Pediatrics* (2003), vol. 112(5):e414

4 D. Ludwig, 'Dietary glycaemic index and regulation of body weight', *Lipids* (2003), vol. 38(2):117–21

5 L. Kucek, et al., 'Grounded guide to gluten: How modern genotypes and processing impact wheat sensitivity', *Comprehensive Reviews in Food Science and Food Safety* (2015), vol. 14:285–302

6 K. Heaton, et al., 'Particle size of wheat, maize and oat test meals: Effects on plasma glucose and insulin responses and on the rate of starch digestion in vitro', *American Journal of Clinical Nutrition* (1988), vol. 47:675–82

7 E. Cheraskin, 'The breakfast/lunch/dinner ritual', *Journal of Orthomolecular Medicine* (1993), vol. 8(1):6–10

8 J.T. Braaten, et al., 'High beta-glucan oat bran and oat gum reduce postprandial blood glucose and insulin in subjects with and without type 2 diabetes', *Diabetic Medicine* (1994), vol. 11(3):312–18

9 M.S. Bray and M.E. Young, 'Circadian rhythms in the development of obesity: Potential role for the circadian clock within the adipocyte', *Obesity Reviews* (2007), vol. 8(2):169–81. See also S. Taheri, et al., 'Short sleep duration is associated with reduced leptin, elevated ghrelin, and increased body mass index', *PLoS Medicine* (2004), vol. 1(3):e62

Chapter 12

1   C. Vandenberghe, et al., 'Caffeine intake increases plasma ketones: An acute metabolic study in humans', *Canadian Journal of Physiology and Pharmacology* (2017), vol. 95(5):445–58

2   X. Jiang, et al., 'Coffee and caffeine intake and incidence of type 2 diabetes mellitus: A meta-analysis of prospective studies', *European Journal of Nutrition* (2014), vol. 53(1):25–38

3   X. Shi, et al., 'Acute caffeine ingestion reduces insulin sensitivity in healthy subjects: A systematic review and meta-analysis', *Nutrition Journal* (2016), vol. 15:103

4   M.S. Beaudoin, et al., 'Caffeine ingestion impairs insulin sensitivity in a dose-dependent manner in both men and women', *Applied Physiology, Nutrition, and Metabolism* (2013), vol. 38(2):140–7

5   L.L. Moisey, et al., 'Caffeinated coffee consumption impairs blood glucose homeostasis in response to high and low glycaemic meals in healthy men', *American Journal of Clinical Nutrition* (2008), vol. 87(5):1254–61

6   K. Liu, et al., 'Effect of green tea on glucose control and insulin sensitivity: A meta-analysis of 17 randomised controlled trials', *American Journal of Clinical Nutrition* (2013), vol. 98(2):340–8

7   X. Wang, et al., 'Effects of green tea or green tea extract on insulin sensitivity and glycaemic control in populations at risk of type 2 diabetes mellitus: A systematic review and meta-analysis of randomised controlled trials', *Journal of Human Nutrition and Dietetics* (2013), vol. 27(5):501–502

8   A. Alkerwi, et al., 'Daily chocolate consumption is inversely associated with insulin resistance and live enzymes in the observation of cardiovascular risk factors in Luxembourg study', *British Journal of Nutrition* (2016), vol. 115(9):1661–8

9   C.E. Marsh, et al., 'Consumption of dark chocolate attenuates subsequent food intake compared with milk and white chocolate in postmenopausal women', *Appetite* (2017), vol. 116:544–51

Chapter 13

1   'Scientific Opinion on the substantiation of health claims related to konjac mannan (glucomannan) and reduction of body weight'
    EFSA Journal 2010;8(10):1798 – see www.efsa.europa.eu/en/efsajournal/pub/1798

2   R. Kurzweil and T. Grossman, *Transcend: Nine Steps to Living Well Forever*, New York: Rodale, 2010.

Recommended Reading

Patrick Holford & Jerome Burne, *The Hybrid Diet*, Piatkus (2018)

Patrick Holford, *The Low-GL Diet Bible*, Piatkus (2009)

Patrick Holford & Fiona McDonald Joyce, *The Low-GL Diet Cookbook*, Piatkus (2005)

Patrick Holford & Kate Staples, *Burn Fat Fast*, Piatkus (2013)

Resources

Hybriddiet.co.uk

The website www.hybriddiet.co.uk provides support material for this book and *The Hybrid Diet*. You'll also find information on our worldwide seminars, webinar and retreats, plus products and services that can support you on the 5-Day Diet.

100% Health Check

You can have your own personal health and nutrition assess-ment online using Patrick Holford's 100% Health Check. This gives you a personalised assessment of your current health, and what you most need to change, including a metabolic check to gauge your risk of metabolic syndrome, and a BioAge Check. Visit www.patrickholford.com and go to 'FREE health check'.

100% Health Club

If you join the 100% Health Club you'll get a 40-page report after completing the 100% Health Check, and unlimited access to help you address your needs as your health improves. You also receive Patrick Holford's 100% Health newsletter every other month, plus instant access to all past newsletters online; special reports each month, to keep you motivated and informed (and access to his library of hundreds of reports on important health issues); a hotline to use via the private 100% Health members Facebook group; 20 per cent off most seminars and events; up to 30 per cent off all books and supplements from HOLFORDirect. com (up to 15 per cent on foods); and a free copy of a Patrick Holford book on joining. Membership costs £7.99 a month.

The Brain Bio Centre

The Brain Bio Centre is an outpatient clinic of the charitable Food for the Brain Foundation in London, which specialises in the nutritional treatment of mental health issues, ranging from depression and insomnia to Alzheimer's and Parkinson's disease, under the direction of Patrick Holford. The Centre's team of expert nutritional therapists, backed up by a psychiatrist and neurologist, work with you to identify any nutritional and biochemical imbalances that may be contributing to your symptoms, and the consultation provides you with a tailored programme to correct these issues and restore your health. Through a process of nutritional and psychiatric assessment, and appropriate clinical tests, dietary advice and/or supplements will then be recommended. Visit www.brainbiocentre. com or phone: +44 (0)20 8332 9600.

The Food for the Brain Foundation

The Food for the Brain Foundation is a non-profit educational charity, founded by Patrick Holford, which aims to promote awareness of the link between learning, behaviour, mental health and nutrition; and to educate and provide educational material to children, parents, teachers, schools, the public, the catering industry, health professionals and the government. The website has a free Cognitive Function Test. It takes 15 minutes to complete. Depending on your score, it tells you what to do to improve your memory. For more information visit www. foodforthebrain.org

The Institute for Optimum Nutrition
The Institute for Optimum Nutrition (ION), founded by Patrick Holford, offers a three-year diploma course in nutritional therapy. Visit www.ion.ac.uk, address: Ambassador House, Paradise Rd, Richmond TW9 1SQ, UK; phone: +44 (0)20 8614 7815

Find a Nutritional Therapist
BANT, the British Association for Nutrition and Lifestyle Medicine, is the official register of qualified nutritional therapists. You can search for a therapist by area and see their specialisms should you need support with your health issues. See www.bant.org.uk

We train nutritional therapists to support clients, so it is worth asking them if they are up to speed on the Hybrid Diet (which the 5-Day Diet is based on) – details at www. hybriddiet.co.uk

In Ireland see the Nutritional Therapists of Ireland at www.ntoi.ie

5-Day Diet Retreats
Go keto, detox and rejuvenate with Patrick Holford, following his 5-Day Diet, then two days low GL at his Fforest Barn Mountain Retreat in South Wales. These 7-day 'Hybrid Fast Detox Retreats' happen twice a year, in May and September. For details on the next retreats visit www.patrickholford.com/events.

5-Day Diet Delivered to your Door
The Pure Package offer Patrick Holford's diets delivered pre-made to your door for maximum convenience. The 5-Day

Diet Plan gives you all the foods, drinks and supplements. The Pure Package also offer Patrick Holford's Brain Food Plan, which provides daily delicious meals that are low-GL and high in all brain support nutrients. This is a perfect follow-up to the 5-Day Diet. For more details visit www.purepackage.com

Supplements

Patrick Holford has formulated a range of supplements to support optimal health. The backbone of a supplement programme is an optimum multivitamin and mineral, with extra vitamin C and essential fats, both omega-3 and 6. These are provided in the Optimum Nutrition Pack. If over 50, the enhanced version, the 100% Health Pack, provides extra antioxidants.

Cinnachrome® provides Cinnulin®, a potent extract of cinnamon, with 200mcg of chromium which contributes to normal nutrient metabolism and to the maintenance of normal blood glucose levels.

Carboslow® is a source of super-soluble glucomannan fibre, a highly soluble plant fibre that fills the stomach to give a feeling of satiety. Glucomannan contributes to weight loss as part of a calorie-restricted diet. This effect is obtained with a daily intake of 3g glucomannan in three doses of 1g each, together with 1–2 glasses of water before meals. Glucomannan also contributes to the maintenance of normal blood cholesterol levels with a daily intake of 4 grams. In the US and Canada, PGX® is the leading super-soluble fibre that supports weight loss, blood sugar control and satiation.

Get Up & Go® and **Get Up & Go with CarboSlow®**
This is a delicious breakfast shake which is a combination

of vitamins, minerals, essential fats, protein and fibre, and designed to be mixed into a tasty shake. One serving is just 8 GLs and is perfect for those following a low-GL, slow-carb diet.

Get Up & Go with Carboslow provides 1 gram of gluco-mannan with each serving – see above. Served with carb-free milk (such as almond) and a small handful of berries, it is only 4.5 GLs.

There is no need to take a multivitamin and mineral in the morning if you have Get Up & Go since it provides optimal level of all vitamins and minerals. If your multi is twice a day, do take the second dose pm.

GL Support is a combination of Garcinia Cambogia, 5-HTP and chromium. GL Support may be particularly useful for those following a diet or exercise plan. Chromium contributes to normal nutrient metabolism and to the maintenance of normal blood glucose levels. Garcinia Cambogia, a natural source of HCA (see page 98), may contribute to weight management and healthy appetite control. GL Support also contains B vitamins that help energy metabolism and contribute to a reduction in tiredness and fatigue, including vitamin B6, which contributes to normal protein and glycogen metabolism.

Hybrid Support Nutrients Pack combines all the nutrients you need in either a high fat, 5-Day Diet or slow-carb phase for optimal metabolic efficiency.

Ketofast® is a pure form of C8 oil, the most effective MCT oil. Each tablespoon provides 15ml of pure C8 derived from coco-nut oil, without any additives. Each bottle provides 30 × 15ml servings, a month's supply.

All Patrick Holford products are available from good health food shops and direct from www.HOLFORDirect.com or call 0370 3341575. HOLFORDirect also supply a **5-Day Diet Combo,** which provides all the supporting nutrients needed to ensure maximum effectiveness of the programme. The bundle includes: the Hybrid Pack, Ketofast, GL Support with Carnitine, Get Up & Go with Carboslow, Carboslow Powder and ImmuneC High Strength Powder. See www.holfordirect.com/5-day-diet-combo.html

Blessed Herbs Digestive Stimulator is available online from a number of suppliers, or ask in your health food store.

Foods & Other Products
Drop of Life olive oil, high in polyphenols – available from www.holfordirect.com
Organic Seaweed Crispies – available from Clearspring www.clearspring.co.uk
Classic Mild Kimchi – available from Eaten Alive www.eatenalive.co.uk
Engevita Nutritional Yeast with B12 – available from good health food stores and Amazon.
BlueberryActive and **CherryActive** – available from www.holfordirect.com and in health food stores.
Nibble Protein Lemon with Coconut – available from www.nibbleprotein.com
Meridian almond butter (1kg tub) – available from www.meridianfoods.co.uk.

Most health food shops can get these products for you if you ask.

Epsom salts, using the highest-grade salt from carefully-selected sustainable sources – a 100 per cent natural, organic product, free from artificial colours, perfumes and other additives – are available from newton-wood.co.uk. Use the promo code PH10 for a 10 per cent discount.

Glucose and Ketone Testing

Ketoscan Mini measures breath ketones. You can use it as often as you like (and others can too). However, after 300 tests you'll need to buy a new cartridge, which costs £39 at the time of writing. You can buy from ketoscanmini.co.uk using the code PH20 for a £20 discount.

Ketonix® breath analyser measures breath ketones. You can use it as often as you like (and others can too). The tubular device has two parts – the device and a battery part that you charge up then attach so you can use it away from a power source. Alternatively, you can connect it directly to your computer through a USB port. Normally it costs around £168 but, at the time of writing, if you use the code HYBRID you will get 10 per cent off (price is set in dollars). Go to www.ketonix.com/hybrid.

Keya Smart is a simple to use but state of the art monitor for testing glucose and ketones at the same time from a pin prick of blood that is fed onto a strip inserted into the monitor. It then records and shows you your ketone and glucose level and records all results so you can see your trends. The best deal is to get the 'KEYA® Smart Meter Kit + 3 vials' which gives you 110 test strips, each providing a combined Glucose-Ketone test. That's enough for a month's worth of testing, three times a day. The pack includes the premium colour touchscreen meter, lancing device, 25 lancets, micro-USB cable, wall charger, carry case, control solution, quick start guide and instruction booklet. At the time of writing it costs £189. It is easy to use and the instruction booklet explains everything very clearly. Go to www.keyasmart.com. The cost of strips, when you need more, works out much cheaper than monitors that require different strips for glucose and ketones.

Other Tests

HbA1c and IgG food intolerances: YorkTest Laboratories have self-test kits for HbA1c (glycosylated haemoglobin) called Diabetes Check, which is the best measure of your blood sugar status. Use the code PH10 to get £10 off. They also have a self-test kit for identifying food intolerances, called Food Scan. The FoodScan 113 identifies the foods causing the intolerance and the level of intolerance. In addition, the service includes nutritionist consultations and comprehensive support and advice on managing your elimination diet. To order call YorkTest Laboratories on 0800 130 0580 or visit www.yorktest.com. Use the code PH50 to get £50 off.

Index

(Page numbers in *italic* refer to diagrams; **bold** to recipes)

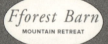